Evaluating Health Promotion:
Practice and Methods

Evaluating Health Promotion:
Practice and Methods

· ·

Edited by
Margaret Thorogood
and
Yolande Coombes
London School of Hygiene and Tropical Medicine

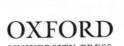

OXFORD
UNIVERSITY PRESS

OXFORD

UNIVERSITY PRESS

Great Clarendon Street, Oxford OX2 6DP

Oxford University Press is a department of the University of Oxford.
It furthers the University's objective of excellence in research, scholarship,
and education by publishing worldwide in

Oxford New York

Athens Auckland Bangkok Bogotá Buenos Aires Cape Town
Chennai Dar es Salaam Delhi Florence Hong Kong Istanbul Karachi
Kolkata Kuala Lumpur Madrid Melbourne Mexico City Mumbai Nairobi
Paris São Paulo Shanghai Singapore Taipei Tokyo Toronto Warsaw

with associated companies in Berlin Ibadan

Oxford is a registered trade mark of Oxford University Press
in the UK and in certain other countries

Published in the United States
by Oxford University Press Inc., New York

© Oxford University Press, 2000

The moral rights of the author have been asserted
Database right Oxford University Press (maker)

First published 2000
Reprinted 2001

A catalogue record for this book is avalable from the British Library
Data available

Library of Congress Cataloging in Publication Data
Evaluating health promotion : practice and methods / edited by
Margaret Thorogood and Yolande Coombes.
p. cm.
Includes index.
0 19 263169 1
1. Health promotion—Evaluation. I. Thorogood, Margaret.
II. Coombes, Yolande.
[DNLM: 1. Health Promotion—standards. 2. Program Evaluation-
-methods. WA 590 E915 2000]
RA427.8.E95 2000 613'.068—dc21 99-39416
ISBN 0 19 263169 1

Typeset by Bibliocraft, Dundee
Printed in Great Britain
on acid-free paper by
Bookcraft (Bath) Ltd
Midsomer Norton, Avon

Foreword

....

This book could scarcely be more opportune. 'Health Promotion', focusing largely on individuals, families and on local communities, burgeoned in the 1980s and 1990s, but became somewhat detached from the rest of Public Health. During those years health promotion was at best marking time, its main intellectual basis in the social, economic, environmental, determinants of health rejected by a dominant government.

The Health Promotion movement grew from Public Health, its personal health services for example and from modern epidemiology with its demonstration of the salience of personal lifestyles and risk factors. But Health Promotion enriched this with insights, data and methods from psychology, sociology and anthropology, from education, and with communication skills. Now with a different government philosophy and agenda there's a return to a more rational comprehensive view of the potential for improving the people's health.

As I write (August 1999) I've just received the Chief Medical Officer's regular 'update' sent to all doctors. The first item is a detailed account of *Saving Lives: Our healthier nation*, the strategy whitepaper for improving health and against inequality. This involves a 'three-way partnership' of Government—joined up across departments, local organisations, and individuals.

Evaluating Health Promotion, from the Health Promotion Research Unit at the London School, indicates how far and how deep this latest front of Public Health has reached.

The book consists of opening and closing integrative chapters by the editors, and an historical overview, classical and contemporary, including a 'history of evaluation' itself.

Half the book is devoted to methods of evaluation. These accounts without exception are hard-headed and practical, manifestly arising from the authors' own experience. Chapter headings indicate the range: combining the qualitative and quantitative (with an interesting conclusion on a social-ecology approach); experimental designs (the randomised controlled trial and alternatives); the role of focus groups (illuminating also on 'social marketing'); economic evaluation (convincingly arguing the case against common scepticism); the evaluation of process (as distinct from outcome); and the use of risk factor simulation models (enabling comparison of gains from different interventions).

Next are four illustrations of evaluations in practice—using mass media, community development initiatives, the problems in clinical settings (the main one, it tactfully hints, being the health professionals), and, unexpectedly, evaluating the dissemination of health promotion research.

I am glad to commend this book throughout Public Health and Health Promotion, and hopefully to clinical colleagues as well. These will be involved, in the education of patients for example—*Saving Lives* is catagoric here. The scope for Health Promotion and its particular contribution is set to grow. Consider a single example. Exercise, physical activity, is one of our serious national health failures: a well-informed population engaging unequally (of course), but highly and less educated, affluent and poor, all of them too little. And the need, if anything, increases, viz the epidemic of overweight/obesity and the emergent 'anti-ageing' movement. It will need all our efforts to alter environmental structures, social norms, and people's behaviour.

JN Morris
Emeritus Professor of Public Health
Department of Public Health and Policy
London School of Hygiene and Tropical Medicine

Contents

....

Contributors

....

Health Promotion Research Unit, Department of Public Health and Policy, Keppel Street, London WC1E 7HT.

Salah Al-Zaroo, Director, Department of Continuing Education, University Graduates Union, PO Box 45, Hebron, West Bank, formerly Research Fellow, Health Promotion Research Unit.

Sarah Basham, General Practitioner, formerly Visiting Research Fellow, Health Promotion Research Unit.

Virginia Berridge, Professor of History, Health Promotion Research Unit.

Patrick Branigan, Research Fellow, Health Promotion Research Unit.

Annie Britton, Lecturer, Health Promotion Research Unit and Cancer and Public Health Unit.

Yolande Coombes, Honorary Lecturer, Health Promotion Research Unit. Address for correspondence: PO Box 529, Blantyre, Malawi.

Dominique Florin, Honorary Lecturer, Health Promotion Research Unit. Address for correspondence: King's Fund, 11–13 Cavendish Square, London W1M 0AN.

Rachel Jewkes, Honorary Senior Lecturer, Health Promotion Research Unit. Address for correspondence: CERSA Women's Health, Medical Research Council, Private Bag X385, Pretoria 0001, South Africa.

Jonathan Karnon, Research Fellow, Health Economics Research Group, Brunel University, Uxbridge UB8 3PH.

Gillian Lewando-Hundt, Senior Lecturer, Health Promotion Research Unit.

Wendy Macdowall, Research Fellow, Health Promotion Research Unit.

Kirstin Mitchell, Research Fellow, MRC IES/STD Intervention Trial, PO Box 1603, Masaka, Uganda, formerly Research Fellow, Health Promotion Research Unit.

Bhash Naidoo, Research Fellow, Health Promotion Research Unit.

William Stewart, Research Fellow, Health Promotion Research Unit.

Margaret Thorogood, Reader in Public Health and Preventative Medicine, Health Promotion Research Unit.

Kaye Wellings, Senior Lecturer, Health Promotion Research Unit.

David Wonderling, Research Fellow, Health Promotion Research Unit and Cancer and Public Health Unit.

Part I

....

Overview

1

....

Introduction

Yolande Coombes and Margaret Thorogood

The past two decades have seen major change and development in health promotion. The boundaries of what is described under the heading of health promotion have widened, and the number of people who work in the field of health promotion has increased exponentially. Health promotion has now reached the point where credible demonstrations of the value of its activity and its effectiveness are needed in order to sustain and expand the current position. However, this is being hampered because there are unresolved theoretical and practical issues concerning the evaluation of health promotion, which are still being hotly debated. The purpose of this book is to contribute to that debate; exploring the wide range of evaluation activity, highlighting the theoretical and practical issues, offering examples and suggestions for further development, and pointing a way out of the current, often sterile, arguments.

In this chapter we shall start by discussing some important definitions, and briefly describe some of the issues and questions facing those who want to evaluate health promotion.

What is meant by health?

Before we can begin to discuss what is meant by health promotion, we first need to consider what we mean by the word 'health'. Our health, and how we view it, is subject to personal, social, biomedical, spiritual, emotional, and physical factors, and there is a wide variety of concepts of health, which differ between individuals, between professions, and between cultures. There are many ways of dichotomizing these concepts. One dichotomy which is relevant to the discussion of health promotion is that between the rather negative view of health as the absence of disease and the more positive view of health being defined by the presence of certain attributes. For example, using the former definition, a person might be defined as healthy if they had no symptoms of disease, and no pathology could be detected. This would be a relatively rare situation, since even fit and active people suffer from minor problems and aches and pains. Moreover, it does not accord very well with the common meaning of being healthy or well; an elderly woman with diabetes and chronic bronchitis might still answer a query about her health with 'I'm very well in myself' although she is obviously not without symptoms or pathology. It is also not a helpful definition when desirable goals for either treatment or health promotion are being considered because it is somewhat utopian to expect the total absence of disease. At the other end of the spectrum is a definition of health as complete physical and mental well-being. Again, this is a state which is unlikely ever to be achieved.

There is a danger that health is equated with longevity, especially when seeking ways of measuring health promotion outcomes. Years of life gained, or increase in average life expectancy, are easy to measure, but they do not necessarily equate with health gain. An extra year spent severely disabled following several years of unpleasant treatment would probably not be considered an advantage by many people.

In general, it is more useful to think of health in relative terms, and to bring into the definition the concept of enablement in addition to the concept of well-being. Health should

---

> ## Box 1.1 Definitions of health
>
> Health is the extent to which an individual or group is able, on the one hand, to realise aspirations and satisfy needs; and on the other hand, to change or cope with the environment. (WHO 1984)
>
> A person's optimum state of health is equivalent to the state of the set of conditions which fulfil or enable a person to work to fulfil his or her realistic chosen and biological potentials. Some of these conditions are of the highest importance for all people. Others are variable dependent upon individual abilities and circumstances. (Seedhouse 1986, p. 61)
>
> Health is seen as a resource for everyday life, not the objective of living . . . Health is a positive concept emphasising social and personal resources, as well as physical capabilities. (WHO 1986)

not be considered as a goal in itself, but rather as the condition which allows us to achieve whatever it is that we want to achieve. The meaning of health is dynamic and changes over time and within different contexts. Box 1.1 outlines some different definitions of health that have been applied which highlight this variation in the interpretation of what health is.

What is meant by health promotion?

Health promotion has been defined in many different ways. Less than half a century ago, health promotion meant nothing more than didactic health education. Since then the concept has come of age, and round it has grown the beginnings of a new profession. What we now understand as health promotion includes activities such as public policy aimed at improving health, clinical interventions which aim to prevent disease, education which aims to enable people to take more control of their health, and a variety of interventions which aim to strengthen communities and increase social capital. All of these activities will happily fit within the definition used in the Ottawa Charter for health promotion (WHO 1986), which defined health promotion as 'the process of enabling people to increase control over and to improve their health'. The problem with such a broad definition is that it is often difficult to decide what is, and what is not, health promotion, and there is a danger that energy is wasted arguing about the precise position of the boundaries, rather than concentrating on the common aim of enabling people to have more control over their health, and to be able to live the life they choose.

Health promotion is a relatively new discipline, and not yet fully accepted as such; although the increasing number of academic courses and professional qualifications in health promotion is evidence of its development and suggests that it is gradually becoming more accepted as a discipline in its own right. Further evidence to support this comes from the increased interest in health promotion by governments, and a proliferation in health promotion research. Health promotion has been described as 'paradigmatic of an emerging late modern medicine' (Burrows *et al.* 1995), or as a post-modern discipline characterized by its eclectic nature, and broad range of activities. Others have viewed health promotion as an umbrella term for a collection of activities designed to improve health (Kemm and Close 1995). However one views health promotion, it has developed, broadened, and become more sophisticated in its approach. This, in turn, has complicated the process of evaluation (Nutbeam 1998).

The evaluation of health promotion

Evaluation has become an increasingly important concept. The concepts of efficiency and cost-effectiveness are now central to the development of new initiatives in many spheres, including education and, most of all, health. Associated concepts such as quality assurance and audit have become increasingly important. The powerful Evidence Based Medicine movement, which insists that the randomized controlled trial is the ultimate tool for evaluation gives more weight to the role of treatment than prevention in the debate on the relative effectiveness of the two approaches (Health Promotion International 1996). In defining itself as a new, and separate, discipline, health promotion has attempted to distance itself from curative medicine by focusing on a holistic approach to health (Burrows *et al.* 1995). Yet, if health promotion is to maintain or enhance its position as an important policy option, it must engage credibly with the Evidence Based Medicine movement.

Evaluation means literally to place a value or to quantify the worth. The problem in evaluating health promotion is deciding how to value or quantify the outcome. One of the difficulties facing the evaluation of any health promotion activity is deciding on what value to give to 'health'. We have already discussed the difficulty in defining health, and the fact that the concept of health tends to be a relative one. It is likely, then, that any value placed on health will be subjective and interpreted on an individual basis. It is tempting to only measure outcomes in terms that are easily quantifiable, while ignoring those that cannot be so easily quantified. The danger is that we will measure what is easy to evaluate and ignore what is valuable. This is one of the challenges which faces us in developing useful and meaningful methods of evaluating health promotion. In this book we shall be arguing that it is not enough to simply opt out of evaluating outcomes, and nor is it sufficient to concentrate solely on easily quantifiable outcome measures, such as morbidity or mortality. Most evaluations aim to demonstrate the attribution of an effect, this is most usually done by determining the exact relationship between an intervention and the outcome. Within health promotion, the desire for measurement in terms of an outcome evaluation has meant that outcomes are often defined in vague terms or measured inaccurately or proximally, or are included when it is inappropriate to do so (Green and Lewis 1986). The range of activities involved in health promotion, and the multiple levels of operation, generate difficulties for its evaluation. Each type of activity demands a different form of evaluation. The issue in health promotion evaluation is the accuracy and appropriateness of measurement. This applies equally to quantitative and qualitative study designs. There cannot be just one method for

the evaluation of health promotion initiatives because the
initiatives themselves draw on a variety of methods and disciplines. Unfortunately, the methodologies for evaluation have
sometimes been borrowed uncritically from other, more narrowly defined disciplines. As a consequence, health promotion
has been evaluated using inappropriate tools, leading to un-
sustainable conclusions (Speller *et al.* 1997). The challenge in
the next decade is to develop more accurate and appropriate
measures and tools for the evaluation of a wide range of
different health promotion initiatives (Health Promotion International 1996; Mant 1996; Speller *et al.* 1997).

The importance of process evaluation

Outcome evaluation aims to determine whether there is a
relationship between an activity and the outcome. But there is
another, important, part of health promotion evaluation
which concerns the question of why certain outcomes happen. This is the area of process evaluation. Process evaluation
enables us to explore what is going on within a health promotion initiative, often producing results which are a great
surprise to the researchers! Moreover, process evaluation
can be used iteratively during the process of an intervention
to refine and improve the methods used. Process evaluation
allows the validity of the subjects' viewpoint, and of the
subjects' value system. The Ottawa Charter viewed health
promotion as a process not an outcome, health promotion is
carried out with people not on them.

This book

This book argues for a broad minded approach to developing a toolbox of methods for evaluating health promotion,
which avoids the destructive tendency to sit firmly in one
methodological camp ignoring anything heard coming from
other camps. The next chapter recounts the development of
health promotion, and outlines why an historical approach to

evaluation is important within the policy arena, as well as discussing the recent history of evaluation itself. Part II, on the 'Methods of evaluation', discusses some of the problems and the strengths of different qualitative and quantitative methods. Chapter 3 emphasizes the need to combine both qualitative and quantitative approaches to evaluation and the need for multiple theories and methods for a discipline which is by nature eclectic and broadly focused. Chapter 4 concentrates on experimental designs in health promotion evaluation. Chapters 5, 6, 7, and 8 look at the practicalities of using particular methodologies for the evaluation of health promotion; in turn they examine focus groups, the theoretical and practical problems associated with economic evaluation, process evaluation techniques, and risk factor simulation models. Part III discusses some of the particular issues of putting evaluation into practice. Chapter 9 examines the difficulties inherent in evaluating mass media campaigns, and in particular addresses the difficulties of attribution. Chapter 10 focuses on the problems associated with evaluating community development initiatives, while the relationship between prevention and treatment and the role for health promotion in clinical settings is explored in Chapter 11. Chapter 12 discusses the much neglected need to evaluate the process of disseminating the findings of health promotion research.

Key points

- Health is a subjective concept.
- It is difficult to evaluate health promotion activities because it is difficult measure health.
- Health promotion involves a variety of multi-disciplinary activities; therefore a range of methods for evaluation must be used.
- Rigorous evaluation methods are needed in order to develop a new evidence base for the further development of health promotion.

References

Burrows, R., Bunton, R., Muncer, S., and Gillen, K. (1995). The efficacy of health promotion, health economics and later modernism. *Health Education Research* **10**, 242–9.

Green, L. W. and Lewis, F. M. (1986). *Measurement and evaluation in health education and health promotion*. Mayfield, Palo Alto, CA.

Health Promotion International (1996). Where next for evaluation? *Health Promotion International* **11**, 171–3.

Kemm, J. and Close, A. (1995). *Health promotion. Theory and practice*. Macmillan, London.

Mant, D. (1996). Health promotion and disease prevention: the evaluation of health service interventions. In *Scientific basis of health services* (ed. M. Peckham and R. Smith), pp. 170–8. BMJ Publishing Group, London.

Nutbeam, D. (1998). Evaluating health promotion—progress, problems and solutions. *Health Promotion International* **13**, 27–44.

Seedhouse, D. (1986). *Health: The foundations for achievement*. Wiley, Chichester.

Speller, V., Learmonth, A., and Harrison, D. (1997). The search for evidence of effective health promotion. *British Medical Journal* **315**, 361–2.

WHO (1984). *Health promotion: a discussion document on the concept and principles*. World Health Organisation Regional Office for Europe, Copenhagen.

WHO (1986). *Ottawa charter for health promotion*. World Health Organisation & Health and Welfare, Ontario.

2

....

Historical and policy approaches to the evaluation of health promotion

Virginia Berridge

Using historical approaches to evaluate 'health promotion' might just mean a history of the last twenty or so years. We could start with the 1974 Lalonde Report in Canada, *A new perspective on the health of Canadians,* and trace a subsequent cascade of 'milestones' in health promotion history such as the 1976 policy document, *Prevention and health: everybody's business,* followed by the 1978 declaration of Alma Ata, *Health for all* from WHO in 1981 and its 38 targets for health in the European Region in 1985. The Ottawa Charter for Health Promotion followed in 1986. The Healthy Cities project was launched in 1987. In 1992, came the publication of the *Health of the nation,* while the new British Labour government in 1997 for the first time specifically appointed a minister responsible for what it now termed 'public health'. Further initiatives have followed.

Such parades of dates and policy documents provide a sense of excitement and movement. They encourage us to think that these years have been ones of incessant activity, that progress has been made, that new definitions and concepts have been

established. Health promotion, as other chapters in this vo-
lume demonstrate, is essentially a fuzzy concept—but, for the
purposes of this chapter, it is taken to mean the developments
since the 1980s whereby the issue of individual health in
relation to the environment has made its way in various forms
onto the policy agenda. There is a danger that the parade of
dates fronting this article encourages a type of 'Whig history'
where all events are seen as leading to a time of greater
understanding and action in the present. At a broader level,
these events do little to deepen historical understanding. They
do not tell much about **why** or **how** these policies have
developed. This chapter will develop a historical understanding of 'health promotion' at three different levels. Firstly, it
will look at how what we now term 'health promotion' fits
into changing definitions of public health and the rationales
for those definitions since the eighteenth century. Then it will
examine a more short term form of historical evaluation,
looking at how the 'contemporary history' of recent health
promotion policies can also provide a form of evaluation.
History is a questioning discipline—and so, finally, this chapter
will ask, why are we talking about evaluation at all? What is
the history of the concept of evaluation and why has it now
come centre stage as far as health is concerned?

Level one. The long view: changing definitions of public health since the eighteenth century

Nineteenth century environmentalism

A Health Promotion Glossary commissioned by WHO Europe
defined the 'new public health' of the late twentieth century
in the following terms.

'Professional and public concern with the effect of the total environment in health.
Note The terms build on the old ... public health which struggled
to tackle health hazards in the physical environment. ... It now

includes the socio-economic environment (for example, high unemployment). 'Public health' has sometimes been used to include publicly provided personal health services, such as maternal and child care. The term new public health tends to be restricted to environmental concerns and to exclude personal health services, even preventive ones such as immunization or birth control.' (Draper 1991)

This recent definition is controversial, both for its breadth and for its exclusion of formal health services. Not all would agree with this version. It also evokes a historical legacy— which is perhaps a matter of more general agreement. It takes as its reference point the nineteenth century history of public health, the 'heroic' or 'golden age' which provides, so it is argued, an earlier example of environmentalism in action. The spur to reform was epidemic disease—and especially the impact of cholera outbreaks in 1831–32, 1848, and again in the 1860s. The 'hero' of the period (if we are writing heroic history) was Edwin Chadwick, and his famous *Report on the sanitary condition of the labouring population*, 1842 (Flinn 1965). Chadwick drew the link between dirt and disease, and its association with overcrowding and poor sanitation. He called for better water supplies, drainage, and sewage removal. As a follower of Jeremy Bentham's Utilitarian creed, he saw a strong role for the central state in achieving the greatest good for the greatest number. But Chadwick's practical impact was slight. The Public Health Act of 1848 set up a Central Board of Health. But legislation was only permissive and not compulsory—and there was strong opposition to dictatorship from the centre. Chadwick was removed from his post in 1854 and the Board was abolished. In other industrializing states, however, such conflicts were avoided simply by avoiding the expansion of the central state (Porter 1994).

In Britain, it was at the local level where most was achieved. Sir John Simon, as Medical Officer to the Privy Council Office, helped to push through Public Health Acts in 1872 and 1875 which forced every local authority to establish a sanitary body as well as to inspect housing and monitor food supplies and 'nuisances'. His resignation in 1876 diminished central influence—but local activity still proceeded apace. The Medical Officer of Health (MoH), compulsory for the first time at the local level under the 1875 Act, could be a crucial engine of change (Eyler 1997).

Looking at long term evaluative trends, there are a number of issues to bear in mind about the nineteenth century story. First, the nature of the links between poverty and ill health. Chadwick was Secretary to the Poor Law Commission and his concern for health reform arose out of the concern for pauperism. Ill health caused poverty and therefore a possible reliance on the parish and poor relief. This was the 'human capital' approach to health reform, a response which has often been replicated since. The term 'social capital' in contemporary health promotion recalls this legacy. In the nineteenth century public health reform was a surrogate and replacement for more general social reform (Hamlin 1998).

The question arises of how much impact public health interventions really had? This has been a long running debate among historical demographers which has implications for those who plan and run health services in the contemporary world. The 'McKeown thesis' view that formal medical interventions actually achieved little and rising living standards achieved more has been challenged by a view that gives a greater role to formal public health in the nineteenth century (Lewis 1991; McKeown and Record 1962; Szreter 1988).

It is important to remember, too, how the impetus behind public health was informed by fear. Fear was focused on what was seen as the growth of a 'residuum', a race of degenerates, physically stunted and morally inferior. The residuum was seen as an agent of infection—both of healthy bodies and of the body politic. Dirt was considered to be dangerous at the individual, but also at the political, level. This larger ideological climate for reform was connected with the concern for environmental pollution of the late nineteenth century—the fear of contamination crossed boundaries of social and health concern. It is from this period that we derive our images of the fog shrouded East End of London.

Bacteriology and personal prevention

In the twentieth century the ideology of public health changed and its focus narrowed. Winslow, an American public health authority, identified three phases in the development of public health: the first, from 1840–90, was characterized by environmental sanitation; the second, from 1890–1910, by developments in bacteriology, resulting in an emphasis on isolation and disinfection; and the third, beginning around 1910, by an emphasis on education and personal hygiene, referred to as personal prevention. Take bacteriology first. The discoveries of Koch and Pasteur in the late nineteenth century made public health more important as a profession—it was now possible to pinpoint specific causes of disease, and bacteriology soon came to dominate the public health curriculum. But at another level, these developments moved the focus of attention away from the environment and towards the individual patient as the locus of infection. In fact, some historians have argued that these theories gained widespread acceptability quickly at the political level precisely because they provided such a circumscribed notion of appropriate intervention. At the same time, governments took up the issue of social/ welfare reform through universal education, pensions, health insurance, school meals, and so the barriers between health and social reform became higher and more impermeable.

Some historians and sociologists argue that bacteriology had a negligible effect on the implementation of policy. Its importance lay in preparing the way for the rise of what has been called 'surveillance medicine' (Armstrong 1983). The new public health of the early twentieth century was indeed founded on the concept of 'personal prevention'. This was also a marriage between public health and eugenics. The political imperative for reform was there, especially after the Boer War had revealed the shortcomings of British army recruits and heightened eugenic fears of 'national deterioration' and 'racial decline'. But the focus was on the individual—and especially the individual mother. The concept of 'maternal efficiency' was prevalent. Lewis has pointed to the tensions implicit in the way the infant mortality rate was conceived of as a problem of maternal ignorance (Lewis 1980). The death rate was highest in poor inner city slums, where insanitary living conditions prevailed. Yet public health doctors and civil servants tended to see maternal and child health as a question of providing health visitors, personal services, and health education. Mothers were encouraged to breast feed and to achieve higher standards of domestic hygiene. The possibility of rising living standards and real wages during the First World War may have had more impact on the infant mortality rate, but public health came increasingly to mean the delivery of personal health services.

Running health services in the interwar years

This focus on the personal and the medical ownership of the area meant that what public health doctors did was less distinctive. How did public health doctors differ from general practitioners? The local authority clinic, home of the MoH, seemed to many GPs to be offering only what they could also provide through their individual practices. At the same time, when local government took on the administration of Poor Law hospitals after 1929, many public health doctors found themselves running hospitals. The range of services under the public health umbrella in these interwar years was huge— especially in London, where the municipal hospital system was one of the most extensive in the world. Some argued at the time—and historians have underlined this conclusion— that this administrative expansion was achieved only at the expense of the neglect of the 'community watchdog' role of the MoH (Lewis 1991). Increasingly, the cutting intellectual edge of public health lay outside the discipline—in particular through the work of academics in social medicine, who remained distinct from public health practitioners.

Post war failure and realignment

Public health, contrary to the expectations of many in the profession, did not form the basis of a reformed health service post war. Public health doctors lost their hospital role and faced a decline in clinic work because of the universal access provided to the general practitioner. The local authority role was also under strain with the desire of parts of the public health empire—sanitary inspectors, social workers—to break away. The notion of 'community medicine', of the public health doctor as health strategist, arose at this time. Jerry Morris at the London School of Hygiene and Tropical Medicine first defined the principles of such work as founded in the principles of epidemiology—the community physician would be responsible for 'community diagnosis' and therefore the effective administration of health services. This was the vision put into practice through the policy documents of the late 1960s—the Seebohm Committee and the Todd Commission on Medical Education. Community physicians were to be the lynchpin of the NHS, linking all aspects of lay and medical administration (Lewis 1986). They were to be both advisers and managers. In practice, these roles were difficult to juggle. There were tensions between the responsibility to the community outside the hospital and the accountability to the health authority. After health service reorganization in the 1980s community medicine virtually disappeared.

This is a British story and the detail of these developments were not universally replicated in all countries. Dorothy Porter has pointed out, for example, that industrialization was not a necessary prerequisite for central government intervention in health, nor was the centralization model automatically adopted by states. Forms of public health were clearly dependent on the history and cultures of particular countries (Porter 1994). In general however, changes in the ideology of public health have been similar in both Europe and North America. It is worth stopping at this point briefly to recapitulate some of the themes which emerge from this British focused history and which have relevance to the 'rise of health promotion' in the last quarter century. The public health mandate has narrowed from broad social reform to individual reformation, while the tension between health promotion and preventive activities in the community has often taken second place to a focus on health services and especially their planning and evaluation. Public health personnel/doctors seem to have fallen more readily into the technician–manager rather than the community watchdog role. The relationship with the structures of clinical medicine—as public health has become a medical profession—has been an additional complicating factor.

Level two. The contemporary history of health promotion policies

So this leads us naturally into the second level of historical evaluation, the rationale behind the emergence of a new variant of public health called health promotion. Here the post war shift from infectious to chronic disease as a major cause of ill health and mortality led to an increased emphasis on prevention. But prevention was not an environmental issue, rather a question of remedying defects in individual lifestyle. The rise of this style of thinking can be traced both internationally and nationally, through, for example the 1974 Lalonde report (Lalonde 1974). Many countries followed in publishing similar prevention oriented documents and there was a rapid growth of interest in preventive medicine and in health promotion. The roots of this reorientation can be traced to the research in the 1940s and 1950s which linked smoking with the rise in lung cancer. These scientific 'discoveries', so historians have argued, represented a fundamental paradigm shift in scientific 'ways of knowing'. For biomedical theories of direct causation they substituted the epidemiological notion of relative risk and statistical correlation (Brandt 1990). Within the discipline of statistics, biometrics gave place to public health epidemiology. Epidemiology became the new public health/preventive discipline par excellence, associated with a whole host of health issues, from alcohol and smoking through to diet and heart disease. This was the epitome of the surveillance society. A public health agenda emerged in the 1960s and 1970s which was based on individual avoidance of risk. It developed a strong economic dimension (the 'human capital' arguments of the nineteenth century revisited), and a focus on education of the individual. Consequently the role of health education assumed new significance together with the use and development of techniques of mass persuasion in the health area.

Criticism of this approach came from a variety of directions. Some saw the emphasis on individual responsibility for health as a political ploy to divert attention from the real socioeconomic causes of disease and the failures of health care systems (Tesh 1981). These condemned the 'victim blaming' and 'sickness as sin' arguments implicit within preventive medicine. The individual responsibility argument divorced the person from the social environment. This type of argument was demonstrated by the increasing focus in anti-smoking campaigns on the role of women as mothers (a classic historic public health theme). A naked smoking mother was portrayed in Saatchi and Saatchi advertisements of the 1970s. Mothers were condemned, via epidemiological research, for the low birth weights of their babies, and even for the reduced attainment of their children in later life. There was little sensitivity to the cultural and social realities of life for many women.

Criticism came also from an entirely different direction— from the 'Radical Right', which argued that government wished to institute what it called the 'nanny state' where habits which should be left to individual discretion were regulated and controlled unnecessarily (Le Fanu 1994). Proponents of this line of argument often called attention to the fragility of the scientific arguments supporting particular preventive policies. Prevention was crucially about the reduction of statistical risk to the community as a whole, not, as in curative medicine, about delivering benefits to identifiable individuals. In surveys where the public ranked different medical and health interventions, medical technology ranked high while lifestyle efforts received lower levels of public support.

In the post-war years it was the smoking issue which most clearly epitomized the reorientation of public health towards individual lifestyle. By the 1970s, anti-smoking interests had developed a policy agenda which focused on economic argument (price and tax rises, anti-industry) and on the media (advertising bans, mass media campaigns), sustained through the techniques of epidemiology (Berridge 1998). In the 1980s, the development of AIDS as an issue also epitomized many of those public health concerns. AIDS was a syndrome initially defined solely via epidemiology and through the concept of risk. In the debate on how to respond to the potential epidemic, the old punitive responses of public health to infectious disease—quarantine and notification—were explicitly rejected, often on the advice of historians. AIDS was an epidemiological syndrome par excellence; and it also seemed to exemplify the key tenets of the new public health, stressing individual behaviour modification and individual responsibility rather than any collective reaction (Berridge 1996; Leichter 1991). In the policy responses favoured by western liberal democracies—behaviour modification and health education campaigns—it exemplified the tenets of health promotion.

Recently, a new variant of health promotion has emerged, allied to the 'new environmentalism'. Again the precise meaning and content is unclear. The global environment is involved, but also a redefinition and expansion of risk at the level of the individual in society, the concept of the 'environmental citizen', a rational consumer protecting him or herself from environmental risks (Petersen and Lupton 1996). Health promotion/public health seems to exemplify a new environmental individualism, epitomized by the emergence of the concept of passive smoking, which gave the epidemiological concept of risk an environmental dimension, but one still rooted in the control of individual behaviour and with a strong moral component. Environmentalism at the level of the city or the locality means essentially control of the individual, as for example through the concept of 'community safety' and its elaboration in drug and alcohol free spaces. Reforming environmentally damaging social activities is a major thrust of this new health promotion environmentalism.

Level three. The history of evaluation

So far we have looked at the meaning of historical analysis in the evaluation of health promotion. But we can also turn the issue on its head and ask—why are we talking about evaluation at all? If we went back say thirty or forty years, not only would we not be talking about 'health promotion' as a concept, we would not be thinking of evaluation as one either. Evaluation is also a historically contingent concept and activity. Why is it now so important? To answer that question would take longer than current space allows—and in fact, no contemporary history of evaluation has been written. A few salient issues can briefly be sketched in. Clearly the rise and reorientation of statistical thinking in the post-war years—through epidemiology and the randomized controlled trial—provided an important mindset for this type of approach. Another strand came via the US 'war on poverty' programmes of the 1960s and, in developing countries, via donor funded primary health care initiatives. For both, evaluation had political value in demonstrating 'what worked' and in providing the rationale for further funding. In Britain, a key text so far as health services were concerned was Archie Cochrane's 1971 book *Effectiveness and efficiency*, which presented powerful arguments for the widespread use of the randomized controlled trial in health services. This, he felt, would open up 'a new world of evaluation and control which will, I think, be the key to a rational health service' (Cochrane 1971). Cochrane's specific arguments need to be set in the context of changes in research policy in the 1970s in Britain. The Rothschild 'customer/contractor' reforms in the funding of research by government departments saw much greater potential government planning of research and control over what researchers did. In the health field, the emergence of the evidence-based medicine movement in the 1980s used primarily statistical and economic techniques to decide if interventions were effective. Such approaches were at the basis of the NHS Research and Development programme launched in the 1980s. Increasingly, these arguments were applied across the health arena to preventive as well as curative interventions. The methodology of the randomized controlled trial, increasingly synonymous with 'evidence' (as if there were no other forms of evidence) in health services, began to be advocated for health promotion interventions. The technique, originally used in medicine to evaluate the use of new drugs, spread to preventive interventions in areas such as smoking. Many researchers were uneasy about its inexorable rise, citing its origins in the disciplines of the natural and biological sciences and doubting its universal applicability to programmes as opposed to treatments. Underpinning all these developments was the belief, disputed by some, that rationality could be achieved in health policy. Evaluation and evidence-based policy assumed a depoliticized and atomized health arena. Evaluations rarely incorporated the activities of central government.

Historical evaluation

Historical evaluation of health promotion, as should be clear from this brief survey, does not set out to give some of the answers traditionally associated with the process of evaluation. It cannot tell us what works best, what is cost effective, which intervention to put in place, or advise us on the best technique for assessment. There are no reproducible models for action. Rather, this chapter has tried to point out how health promotion is the latest variant of a public health history which traces its origins to the desire of states to deal with issues of social order and control. It has examined, too, how its current ideology has developed out of the changes in public health concepts which have taken place since the nineteenth century and how these have essentially reflected the perceived role of the state in relation to intervention in social issues. For health promotion currently to call on an idealized nineteenth century lineage without understanding the rationales for that past—and for its own role in the present—is a largely worthless form of historical evaluation. If history does have evaluative 'lessons' it is that public health and its remit have been dependent on the changing framework of state intervention since the nineteenth century and that increasingly, despite appeals to a heroic past, such activities have been narrower and more circumscribed in their remit.

Key points

- The mandate of public health has redefined itself since the nineteenth century—from environmentalism to personal prevention, to running health services, and on to the focus on individual lifestyle and 'risk'.

- Such redefinitions have been inextricably connected with changes in the perceived role of the state and the nature and forms of social order.

- The new environmentalism of contemporary health promotion can be seen as a type of environmental individualism, a refocusing of the lifestyle arguments to encompass sites of risk.

- The notion of 'evaluation' itself in relation to medicine, health, and latterly health promotion is historically contingent and needs historical analysis.

- Using 'golden age' history as a form of support mechanism for contemporary policy risks misunderstanding both past and present. Historical analysis, used in a less partisan way, can help in assessing current ideologies and policies.

References

Armstrong, D. (1983). *Political anatomy of the body. Medical knowledge in Britain in the twentieth century.* Cambridge University Press.

Berridge, V. (1996). *AIDS in the UK: the making of policy 1981–1994.* Oxford University Press.

Berridge, V. (1998). Science and policy; the case of post war smoking policy. In *Ashes to Ashes; the history of smoking and health* (ed. S. Lock, L. Reynolds, and E. M. Tansey), pp. 143–63. Rodopi, Amsterdam.

Brandt, A. (1990). The cigarette, risk and American culture. *Daedalus*, **Fall issue**, 155–76.

Cochrane, A. (1971). *Effectiveness and efficiency. Random reflections on health services.* Nuffield Provincial Hospitals Trust.

Draper, P. (1991). *Health through public policy: the greening of public health*. Greenprint, London.

Eyler, J. (1997). *Sir Arthur Newsholme and State Medicine, 1885–1935*. Cambridge University Press.

Flinn, M. W. (1965). *Report on the sanitary condition of the labouring population of Great Britain by Edwin Chadwick 1842*, edited with an introduction by M. W. Flinn., Edinburgh University Press.

Hamlin, C. (1998). *Public health and social justice in the age of Chadwick. Britain, 1800–1854*. Cambridge University Press.

Lalonde, M. (1974). *A new perspective on the health of Canadians*. Department of National Health and Welfare, Ottawa.

Le Fanu, J. (1994). *Preventionitis. The exaggerated claims of health promotion*. Social Affairs Unit, London.

Leichter, H. (1991). *Free to be foolish. Politics and health promotion in the United States and Great Britain*. Princeton University Press.

Lewis, J. (1980). *The politics of motherhood. Child and maternal welfare in England, 1900–1939*. Croom Helm, London.

Lewis, J. (1986). *What price community medicine?* Harvester, Brighton.

Lewis, J. (1991). The origins and development of public health in the U.K. In *The Oxford textbook of public health* pp. 23–4 (ed. W. Holland *et al.*), Oxford University Press.

McKeown, T. and Record, R. G. (1962). Reasons for the decline of mortality in England and Wales during the nineteenth century. *Population Studies*, **xvi**, 94–122.

Petersen, A. and Lupton, D. (1996).*The new public health. Health and self in an age of risk*. Sage, London.

Porter, D. (1994). *The history of public health and the modern state*. Rodopi, Amsterdam.

Szreter, S. (1988). The importance of social intervention in Britain's mortality decline, c.1850–1914: a reinterpretation of the role of public health. *Social History of Medicine*, **1**(1), 1–37.

Tesh, S. (1981). Disease, causality and politics. *Journal of Health Politics, Policy and Law*, **6**(3), 369–90.

Part II

Methods of evaluation

3

....

Combining quantitative and qualitative approaches to evaluation

Yolande Coombes

Introduction

One of the current debates in health promotion, highlighted in Chapter 1, is the relative value of quantitative and qualitative approaches to evaluation. The debate centres around both theoretical and practical issues as to the merits of the two approaches. It is not possible to resolve all these issues within this anthology, let alone within a single chapter, but within this chapter I shall discuss some of the ways that these issues can be approached and resolved. It has been suggested that quantitative and qualitative approaches should be combined. This has not been suggested in order to reach a peaceful but unsatisfactory compromise, but rather because the unique nature of health promotion interventions *need* evaluation methodologies which utilize both qualitative and quantitative approaches.

This chapter begins by analysing the need for different methodological approaches to evaluation; it then looks at the ways in which qualitative and quantitative approaches can be combined before finally looking at a social ecological approach to health promotion which addresses some of the issues that have been raised.

Reigning supremacy—quantitative or qualitative?

Health promotion is a particularly multi-disciplinary activity—the different disciplines contributing to this book and other health promotion volumes are testament to this. It is partly because of these different contributing disciplines and the varied approaches that each discipline has to evaluation and research that the quantitative versus qualitative debate has arisen. This is an extension of a debate which has been going on in the social sciences for some time. Some strands of this debate will never be resolved; for example it is futile to discuss whether qualitative or quantitative methods are superior, and aspects of the debate such as these rest on a false dichotomy and should be abandoned. This false dichotomy has been exemplified by McKinlay (1993, p. 116) who points out:

All of us in the business of health promotion bring different tools to do the job ... Imagine the patent absurdity of comparing the intrinsic contribution of each of these occupations; or enquiring as to whether a tool like a wrench is more useful and reliable than a paint brush ... But to compare a case study to a randomized controlled trial is to compare wrenches with brushes.

It is obvious for which jobs we would use a paintbrush and for which we need the wrench, but it is at this point that the metaphor with respect to health promotion breaks down. The fundamental problem underlying the qualitative versus quantitative debate in health promotion arises out of collective *certainty* and at the same time *ambiguity* as to which are the appropriate tools to use. Some argue that quantitative methods are the most appropriate, while others argue for qualitative insight. Moreover, further confusion is introduced because these methods are often used incorrectly or inappropriately. Thus, as Speller *et al.* (1997) conclude, health promotion is often being evaluated with inappropriate tools with the consequence that interventions (and therefore health promotion) are assessed as being not effective.

Even within the quantitative and qualitative camps, methods are used inappropriately and conclusions and inferences are made on spurious or ambiguous evidence. This is often the result of methods being employed by people who do not fully understand the methodology and epistemology that they originate from. Within the quantitative field, a hierarchy of evidence has been established (see Chapter 4), which provides methodological rigour to assessment of results, and thus provides us with insight in our interpretation of those results. Some have wrongly added qualitative methods to the bottom of the hierarchy of quantitative methods, ignoring the fact that qualitative methods are derived from a completely different epistemology and do not seek to answer the same questions as quantitative approaches. Qualitative methods are often only considered when quantitative methods have been ruled out, but as the question will have been framed in a positivist quantitative way, they, too, will be unable to provide the answer (Eakin and Maclean 1992).

If qualitative methods are regarded as an extension of quantitative methods, they will always appear inferior, because they are fundamentally different in their approach to evaluation. For example, if we wanted to compare the reduction in serum cholesterol levels from exercise and from medication, then a randomized controlled trial would be the most effective method of evaluation. A qualitative approach to this would not yield any sensible answer, because the nature of the question calls for a quantitative answer. However, if our question was concerned with long term adherence by the population to the two methods of reducing serum cholesterol levels then qualitative methods would have an extremely important role. We would still need the quantitative measurement of serum cholesterol levels in people following the two different regimes, but it would be qualitative methods which would be able to assess how people felt about the different regimes, and what were the contributing factors to how likely they were to adhere to the different regimes in the long term.

Qualitative methods evaluate fundamentally different questions to quantitative methods, and should never be considered on the same hierarchy or scale as quantitative methods. Quantitative methods can best evaluate *whether* there is a relationship between an intervention and a health outcome, whereas qualitative methods are best placed to assess *why* the relationship exists; thus both approaches are needed. Qualitative approaches are more able to assess the relationship between a health outcome and the context in which it occurs, and the processes by which it occurs, whereas quantitative methods allow us to document the magnitude and scale of the change in health status with precision.

Increasing methodological rigour

Should we develop an index of methods for qualitative approaches to evaluation in health promotion? Although it might be abhorrent to many qualitative researchers to suggest a similar hierarchy as that which has been established in the quantitative field, it is possible to see how some practical guidance over the choice of methods employed might improve the evidence base of qualitative work on the evaluation of health promotion. What is needed is for qualitative researchers within the field of health promotion to take a more pragmatic approach to the explanation and interpretation of research methods. Some basic ground rules for evaluating qualitative methods are needed. For example, guidance could be provided over the types of insight a focus group might offer compared to participant oservation or in-depth interviews. Macdonald (1996) suggests a hierarchy of qualitative methods with the most theory-generating, most valid methods on the top and the more descriptive and less inductive methods below. Health promoters need to know why they should choose one qualitative method rather than another, how to use the method appropriately, and how to read critically and interpret the research done by others.

Health promotion needs to establish methodological rigour and scientific credibility if it is to achieve recognition as a discipline Using the term 'science' does not mean that quantitative methods are viewed as superior to qualitative, rather that there is a need for rigour, and for guidance on how all methods of evaluation are used. Practitioners involved in health promotion have been trained in different disciplines, and there needs to be some mechanism for them to assess the relative merits of both quantitative and qualitative approaches. Researchers from within particular disciplines could do more to further the evidence base for health promotion practice by explaining to practitioners the value of their approach and, more importantly, the boundaries for its appropriate use, rather than focusing their energies on the supremacy of one approach over another.

Some of the relative strengths and weaknesses of particular qualitative and quantitative approaches and their appropriate use are outlined elsewhere in this book, and I will not discuss them here. Instead, I would like to now focus on the issue of whether and how we should combine qualitative and quantitative methods in the evaluation of health promotion interventions.

Is there a role for combined qualitative and quantitative approaches?

As has already been mentioned, qualitative and quantitative approaches are based on different epistemologies. Within health promotion the range of feeder disciplines may share methods in common, but the theory on which they are based can be quite different. Thus one of the main arguments against combining qualitative and quantitative methods is an epistemological one—how can you compare and evaluate your findings when the questions you are asking are from different frameworks, paradigms, or ways of seeing. The answer to this may lie in the discussion raised in Chapter 1. Health itself is multidimensional: we can talk of biological health, physical health, mental health, and spiritual health. To investigate what health is, we must formulate questions from several different approaches to health. In the same way, to evaluate how health can be promoted requires us to formulate our questions from the various approaches that can be taken to promoting health. The questions may be grounded in different epistemologies, and it may be difficult and inappropriate to compare them in any way, but in order for us to evaluate health and health promotion in a meaningful and useful way we should approach the topic from all directions. This implies using both quantitative and qualitative approaches.

McKinlay (1993) suggests that what we need to develop is a concept of 'appropriate methodology' for health promotion. Within this concept, no one method would be rated better than another, but methods would be taken on their appropriateness for the job in hand. Using the example of heart disease, McKinlay suggests that health promotion might focus 'downstream', where interventions would be at the level of surgery or drug therapy. Midstream would be primary and secondary prevention efforts focused on smoking cessation, increased exercise, and other risk factor behaviours. Finally, upstream health promotion might focus on interventions with organizations, communities, and macro-social policies. He suggests that no approach can be viewed as intrinsically more worthwhile than any other as each has a role to play in improving health. McKinlay observes that quantitative methods tend to be used for evaluating downstream activities where the unit of analysis is usually the individual whereas qualitative methods are more appropriate upstream where rigorous experimental control is not always possible within the socio-political environment. McKinlay (p. 116) concludes by saying:

The notion of appropriate methodology emphasises the match between the point or level of an intervention and the most suitable research approach contingent of course on the problem, state of knowledge, availability of resources and so forth. There is no right or wrong best methodological approach: appropriateness to the purpose must be the central concern.

If we frame our definition of health in a positive holistic way, and our concept of health promotion is also framed in this way, then, Macdonald (1996) argues, it is necessary to combine qualitative and quantitative methods to evaluate both intermediate (process) indicators and longer term morbidity and mortality outcomes. Macdonald (p. 172) has argued for four underlying premises to evaluative research based on a broad definition of health promotion:

1. Evaluation values and applies needs assessment methods.
2. Evaluation espouses user involvement in the planning of health care programmes and the take-up of services.
3. Evaluation applies quality assurance procedures in relation to the appropriateness of the intervention and its impact on the quality of life.
4. Evaluation respects the need for audit and evaluation as a means of ensuring effectiveness, efficiency and equity.

He argues that, although using multiple methods is not a new idea, the concept of combining the best qualitative and quantitative methods is. Combining a randomized controlled trial with an ethnographic study or an analytical cohort study with the use of nominal groups will produce more valid and reliable results which will help in programme and intervention evaluation.

This argument is developed further by Hepworth (1997), who argues that too many evaluations have concentrated on a conceptualization of health promotion defined by narrow biomedical approaches and focused on health outcomes. She advocates the need to broaden the health outcomes approach to include social health outcomes, and health development outcomes. To do this will require different evaluation methodologies, drawing on qualitative and quantitative methods. Hepworth suggests that 'the future direction for health promotion evaluation needs to employ a framework that elaborates multiple methodologies and approaches necessary for establishing what relationships exist between morbidity, mortality, health advancement and equity' (p. 237).

In summary, because health has so many facets, and health promotion equally is multi-disciplinary, no one theory or perspective will ever enable us to understand fully the complex processes and activities that contribute to health status. Similarly, no one theory will enable us to develop effective intervention programmes.

Combining methods: the concept of triangulation

If we accept the argument that health promotion is multi-dimensional and therefore needs its own appropriate methodology for evaluation, we must accept the need to use multi-method approaches. The notion of combining qualitative and quantitative methods is not new. Four main ways of integrating methods in health promotion have been described by Steckler *et al.* (1992):

1. Qualitative methods are used to develop quantitative measures; for example focus groups used to develop questionnaire items.
2. Qualitative methods are used to help explain quantitative findings; for example in-depth interviews to find out why compliance in a drug trial was low.
3. Quantitative methods are used to help explain qualitative findings; for example the observation that women are reluctant to participate in exercise is qualified by a survey which reveals that it is older women who participate least.
4. Qualitative and quantitative methods are used together for cross-validation and triangulation; for example Before and After trial for smoking cessation is compared with recordings of advice given, and in-depth interviews with clients pre and post the intervention.

In combining methods, the terms triangulation or mixed methods are often used. Denzin (1989) suggests that triangulation can occur in four main ways. Firstly, there is data triangulation, where different sources of data are examined over different times, space, and from different persons. A second approach is investigator triangulation, where more than one investigator is used to carry out or repeat the research. Third, in theory triangulation, alternative theories are used to explore and explain the same body of data. Finally, methodological triangulation involves triangulation within methods and between methods.

In recent years there has been increasing interest in *data* and *methodological* triangulation in particular and it has become 'axiomatic that a combination of qualitative and quantitative methods should produce the most reliable and valid research results' (Milburn *et al.* 1995, p. 348). Although triangulation may increase the reliability and validity of results, it is important not to confuse this with some type of ultimate or objective 'truth' (Eakin and Maclean 1992). It should always be borne in mind that health is a complex set of physiological, biological, emotional, and behavioural factors, that there never will be a 'true' picture, and that what we are striving towards in our evaluations is a better understanding (breadth and depth) or clearer interpretation of that picture.

Theory triangulation has tended to have been avoided. Related to this avoidance has been the avoidance of the fact that triangulation may yield contradictory findings. However, this is not necessarily a negative outcome. Reflecting on contradictory findings is an important process within evaluation as it may result in a more detailed understanding of both the subject matter and the methods used (Milburn *et al.* 1995). Theory triangulation offers health promotion evaluation a way out of the qualitative versus quantitative stalemate. It purposefully involves appraising the same problem or data with different theories. The process of challenging theories and methodological approaches generates a better understanding. This relates back to the notion of health being a multi-dimensional concept which needs multiple methods to evaluate it.

McLeroy *et al.* (1993) have suggested that in order to evaluate health promotion we should begin with the theory of the problem. By focusing on the problem, the health promoter can then work back using different research methods to understand how the problem is socially produced and maintained. We also need to develop 'intervention theories'— summaries of what we know about the relative success of different intervention strategies with particular populations, or in other words, to develop a strong evidence base for health promotion. It has been suggested that a social ecological approach to health promotion combines the 'theory of the problem' with 'intervention theories'.

The social ecological approach to health promotion

The social ecological approach combines a number of disciplines and is a broad paradigm uniting different areas of research to address the broad definition of health promotion as defined in the Ottawa charter 'the process of enabling people to increase control over and to improve their own health'. Social ecological approaches address the relationships between socio-economic, cultural, political, environmental, organizational, psychological, and biological determinants of health and illness (Stokols *et al.* 1996). The social ecological approach is based on the classic agent–host–environment relationship, but ecological models de-emphasize the agent and focus more on the reciprocal relationship between the three factors. In many ways a social ecological approach is based on the 'old' nineteenth century 'environmentalism' public health approach (see Chapter 2).

Stokols (1996) outlined the core principles of a social ecological approach:

- Ecological analyses characterize environmental settings as having multiple physical, social, and cultural dimensions that can influence a variety of health outcomes, including physical health status, emotional well-being and social cohesion.

- The health promotive capacity of an environment is understood, not simply in terms of the health effects of separate environmental features but as the cumulative impact of multiple environmental conditions; for example the cumulative impact of inadequate housing, unemployment, smoking, and obesity on heart disease.

- Human health is not only influenced by environmental factors but by personal attributes including genetic heritage, psychological disposition, and behavioural patterns.

It is the interplay between people and their settings which is important. The same environmental conditions (for example population density, unemployment, access to health services) may affect individuals in different ways according to their personal attributes. Social ecological analyses are based on systems theory in order to be able to understand the complex relationships that affect an individual's health (for example interdependence, homeostasis, negative feedback, deviation). The relationships between people and their environments are seen as two-way. A simple example might be humans creating pollution through industry, cars, and smoking tobacco, and pollution in turn having an impact on childhood asthma. Thus, the overall predictive value of a social ecological approach is in the assessment of the compatibility between people and their surroundings and its effect on their health status (Stokols 1996). Social ecological approaches draw on multiple disciplines ranging from epidemiology, psychology, and sociology to therapeutic medicine. In addition ecological models view patterned behaviour (either of individuals or aggregated levels) as the main outcome of interest. Box 3.1 summarizes a social ecological approach to health promotion evaluations.

By social validity (Point 6 above), Stokols advocates that health promotion interventions should be:
- economically feasible
- firmly grounded in scientific and epidemiological research
- likely to reach a large section of the *targeted* population
- unlikely to cause adverse side effects
- consistent with community priorities, commitments and needs.

In order to carry out a social ecological approach to health promotion an action-research perspective is advocated whereby a continuous process of interventions and evaluation enable theories to guide the development of the interventions within a reciprocal relationship (Stokols 1996). Five key stages of action are advocated within a social ecological approach (Box 3.2).

A social ecological approach is a continuous approach to the evaluation of health promotion interventions. As more insight is gained, the evidence base is increased, and thus the theory

---

Box 3.1   Guidelines for health promotion on social ecological principles

1. Examine the links between multiple facets of health and well-being and diverse conditions of the socio-physical environment.

2. Consider joint and cumulative influence of intrapersonal and environmental conditions on individual and community well-being.

3. Develop health promotion programs that enhance the fit between people and their surroundings.

4. Focus health promotive interventions on high-impact behavioural and organizational leverage points. Human behaviour occurs in recurring patterns which take place in particular settings—these patterns and settings make ideal 'leverage' points.

5. Design health promotion programs that address interdependencies between the physical and social environment and encompass multiple settings.

6. Integrate multi-disciplinary perspectives in the design of health promotion programmes and use multiple methods to gauge scientific and social validity of interventions.

(Stokols 1996)

---

of the problems can be expanded, and the process of working backwards from the problem begins once more.

Although developed to answer some of the criticisms of previous health promotion interventions which were narrowly focused on particular health outcomes without taking into account the context in which they occurred, there is some concern that the social ecological approach is in fact too broad. One solution to this problem has been to stratify the environment and to present distinct research and action or intervention agendas for each layer (Richard *et al.* 1996). For example, a programme to reduce the burden of heart disease might be stratified by individual, household, worksite, community, media, policy makers, and general population. At each level, or in each setting, the health promotion practitioner would work through the five stages of action (see box).

Box 3.2 **Five stages of action**

1. Identify the health problems using data on prevalence, incidence, and health needs assessment from community perspective.

2. Identify the social, psychological, and biological factors of the problem, and identify the interrelationships among these factors at multiple levels.

3. Identify intervention goals, procedures, and outcomes (including social and economic costs).

4. Compare goals to identified previous effective interventions (taking into consideration their population groups and culture).

5. Identify and understand the organizational, cultural, and community context in which the intervention has to occur.

A social ecological approach is complex yet offers a way forward for health promotion, in that health is viewed in a holistic sense and therefore different methods (both quantitative and qualitative) are needed in order to evaluate the different components of health. The approach includes both the quantitative emphasis on whether relationships exist and the qualitative emphasis on why there is a relationship. Most importantly, a social ecological approach addresses health and health promotion in a holistic way so that the context or environment in which health and health outcomes occur are included in the evaluation.

Key points

- No single theory is adequate for evaluating health promotion because of the multi-dimensional nature of health.

- Quantitative evaluations address whether there is a relationship whereas qualitative evaluations address why there is a relationship—thus both approaches are needed.

- A social ecological approach offers a way of not only combining quantitative and qualitative evaluations, but also of taking into account the socio-cultural processes and context of health outcomes.

References

Denzin, N. K. (1989). Strategies of multiple triangulation. In *The research act: a theoretical introduction to sociological methods* (3rd edition), pp. 234–47. Prentice Hall, New Jersey.

Eakin, J, M. and Maclean, H. M. (1992). A critical perspective on research and knowledge development in health promotion. *Canadian Journal of Public Health*, **83**, Supplement 1, S72–6.

Hepworth, J. (1997). Evaluation in health outcomes research: linking theories, methodologies and practice in health promotion. *Health Promotion International*, **12**(3), 233–8.

Macdonald, G. (1996). Where next for evaluation? *Health Promotion International*, **11**(3), 171–3.

McKinlay, J. B. (1993). The promotion of health through planned socio-political change: challenges for research and policy. *Social Science and Medicine*, **36**(2), 109–17.

McLeroy, K. R., Steckler, A. B., Simons Morton, B. G., Goodman, R. M., Gottlieb, N., and Burdine, J. N. (1993). Social science theory in health promotion: time for a new model? *Health Education Research*, **8**, 305–12.

Milburn, K., Fraser, E., Secker, J., and Pavis, S. (1995). Combining methods in health promotion research: some considerations about appropriate use. *Health Education Journal*, **54**, 347–56.

Richard, L., Potvin, L., Kishchuk, N., Prlic, H., and Green, L. W. (1996). Assessment of the integration of the ecological approach in health promotion programs. *American Journal of Health Promotion*, **10**(4), 318–28.

Speller, V., Learmonth, A., and Harrison, D. (1997). The search for evidence of effective health promotion. *British Medical Journal*, **315**, 361–3.

Steckler, A., McLeroy, K. R., Goodman, R. M., Bird, S. T., and McCormick, L. (1992). Toward integrating qualitative and quantitative methods: an introduction. *Health Education Quarterly*, **19**, 1–8.

Stokols, D. (1996). Translating social ecological theory into guidelines for community health promotion. *American Journal of Health Promotion*, **10**, 282–98.

Stokols, D., Allen, J., and Bellingham, R. L. (1996). The social ecology of health promotion—implications for research and practice. *American Journal of health Promotion*, **10**, 247–51.

4

....

Evaluating interventions—experimental study designs in health promotion

Margaret Thorogood and Annie Britton

Introduction

An experimental study, in which a group of people are exposed to an intervention and then compared with another group who have not been exposed, is a standard method for evaluating effectiveness. There are certain situations in which an experimental approach may not be feasible or appropriate, and observational studies or other methods such as simulation (see Chapter 8 on risk factor simulation models) may be used. However, when possible, well designed, controlled experiments can provide vital evidence on the effectiveness of interventions.

Health promotion researchers have a range of experimental study designs to choose from and in this chapter we describe the features of a randomized controlled trial and discuss the problems which might be encountered in using such trials to evaluate the effectiveness of a health promotion intervention. We go on to describe some alternative types of experimental study design and review some of their strengths and weaknesses in relation to their use in evaluating health promotion interventions.

Experimental research

The idea of testing the effectiveness of a treatment on humans by experimentation has been around for a long time. One elegant experiment was carried out as early as 1747 by a ship's surgeon who was looking for a cure for the scurvy which was then a major man-power problem for the Navy. James Lind describes how he took twelve sailors with scurvy whose cases were *'as similar as I could get them'*. The sailors *'lay together in one place'* and had *'one diet common to all'*. They were assigned, in pairs, six different medications, including vinegar, cider, sea water, 'elixir vitriol', a mixture including garlic and mustard seed amongst other things, and *'each two oranges and one lemon every day'*. The results were dramatic: *'the most sudden and good effects were perceived from the use of the oranges and lemon; one of those who had taken them being at the end of six days fit for duty'* (Lind in Buck *et al.* 1988). This early example of a clinical trial contained many of the aspects that are still important in the design of health care trials today:

- the question to be addressed had important public health implications;
- there was more than one treatment and the effects were compared, that is, the trial was controlled;
- attempts were made to choose patients who were similar and to treat them similarly in all other ways except for the treatment bring compared, that is, the effect of potential confounding factors was controlled;
- the choice of oranges and lemons as a potential cure to be tested was not haphazard, but was based on the observation of non-experimental accounts of scurvy being cured or prevented when citrus fruit was available, that is, the trial represented part of a greater body of work, which included a review of the available evidence.

One thing that is not clear from Lind's experiment is whether the choice of treatment was allocated randomly.

Randomized controlled trials

Confounding factors are variables that are linked both to the intervention and to the observed outcome. These factors, for example age or social class, can distort the relationship between an intervention and outcome. In order to avoid spurious associations, it is important that attempts are made to control for these confounding factors. If people are randomized into groups, then it is likely that any confounding factors, **whether or not** they had been previously identified, will be equally distributed between the groups. Hence any later differences observed between the groups can be attributed with more certainty to the difference in the interventions. The randomization should be done in such a way that neither the researcher allocating the treatment group, nor the person being allocated, can predict in advance which intervention will be allocated. In this way the possibility of a biased allocation on the grounds of willingness to be in one particular group, or perceived potential to gain benefit from one particular intervention, will be eliminated.

In order to reduce further bias, it is preferable that during the trial both the participants and the researcher(s) are unaware as to which intervention or treatment is being given. This is called a **double-blind trial** and is relatively easy to conduct when the active treatment is some kind of drug for which an inactive but visually identical placebo can be prepared. It is much less easy in trials of health promotion interventions.

The unit of randomization is usually an individual; sometimes it is more appropriate or convenient to randomize by clusters, for example all the patients seen by a particular doctor, or by even larger communities, such as small towns. Community randomization is particularly useful when a community-based intervention, for example, a campaign to increase uptake of childhood vaccination, is being tested (although the choice of this method of randomization has implications for the sample size required).

In evidence-based medicine, it is accepted that there is a hierarchy of reliable evidence, with the results of randomized controlled trials (RCTs) or meta-analyses of those trials at the top (see Table 4.1). This hierarchy reflects the degree to which the different study designs may be susceptible to potential selection bias and therefore how certain we can be that the observed effects are actually attributable to the intervention. When randomization is lacking, comparison groups may have important baseline differences, and this threatens the *internal validity* of trial results. However, randomized trials are sometimes criticized for being too restrictive in their recruitment and too remote from normal practice, thus threatening their *external validity* and the generalizability of their findings.

Table 4.1 Heirarchy of experimental research evidence

Level	Source of evidence
I	Well-designed randomized controlled trials
II	Well-designed controlled studies with quasi-randomization
III	Well-designed controlled studies with no randomization
IV	Before and after studies
V	Small case reports or studies with no control group

Source: based on NHS Centre for Reviews and Dissemination, 1996

Ultimately, the value of the evidence depends on how well the study was designed, conducted, analysed, and reported as well as the position of the study design in the methodological hierarchy. Poor quality RCTs are less useful than well-designed non-randomized studies. All study designs need to address issues such as how to deal with subjects who do not comply with the intervention protocol, those who switch to a different intervention, and those who cannot be traced at the follow-up. RCTs have extra considerations, such as acquiring consent from the subjects and deciding at what stage in the study to randomize the subjects (Pocock 1997).

The enthusiasm for randomized trials is upheld by the Cochrane Collaboration, a world-wide network which aims to synthesize the most reliable evidence assessing interventions for prevention, treatment, and rehabilitation of specific health problems into regularly updated systematic reviews. The systematic reviews produced by the Collaboration rely predominantly on evidence from randomized controlled trials and there are now well-documented guidelines for those wishing to prepare such reviews (Chalmers and Altman 1995).

Randomized controlled trials versus non-randomized studies

It is often stated that non-randomized studies report larger estimates of treatment effects than those using random allocation (Schultz *et al.* 1995). This may be particularly true in the evaluation of health promotion interventions where non-randomized studies may include disproportionate numbers of people who have greater capacity to benefit from the intervention. For example, if the intervention is preventive, for example a pap smear to detect early stage cervical cancer, it could be misleading to compare the results of those who volunteer for treatment with those who do not respond to invitations; their baseline risks are unlikely to be the same. This problem can be addressed when the study is being interpreted, by examination of risk profiles or sub-group analysis (but undetected confounding will threaten the internal validity of such studies). However, in a review of 18 papers that compared the results of randomized and prospective non-randomized studies, the non-randomized studies did not give consistently larger estimates of intervention effect (Britton *et al.* 1998). Seven of the 18 papers in the review found that the two study types gave almost identical treatment effect estimates. Of these seven, five had used risk-adjustment techniques in the non-randomized studies for baseline differences, which suggests that rigorous methodology in non-randomized studies gives more valid results than those where confounding is ignored.

The external validity of a randomized controlled trial

RCTs can be criticized because the way that such trials are designed tends to exclude many of those people to whom the results will subsequently be applied. The conditions in which the study was conducted may not represent normal practice or, more importantly, the individuals who participate in such research may be different from the rest of the population. These concerns apply to all study designs, but it is likely that randomized controlled trials suffer the most. Non-randomized studies can utilize existing practice to evaluate different strategies, while randomized controlled trials are more likely to create an artificial situation in which trial inclusion criteria and the intervention administration can be controlled.

A review of 20 published papers which reported entry characteristics of both participants and non-participants (Britton *et al.* 1998) included four trials of interventions aimed at promoting health. In these trials participants were likely to be younger; to be of higher social status (in terms of income, housing, education, or car ownership); and to believe in and adopt a 'healthier lifestyle' (for example non-smoker, take exercise) in comparison to non-participants. Non-participants included those not invited to participate (for example failed to meet the eligibility criteria) and those who refused. Where participants are found to differ from the rest of the population, the generalizability of the study findings should be questioned.

The effect of personal preferences in non-blinded trials

Another problem, relevant to RCTs of health promotion interventions, is that the recipients' preferences for, or beliefs about the effectiveness of, the interventions may influence the outcome. This could cause the results of such trials to be distorted. It is unavoidable that some people will have preferences for one intervention or another and recruitment to randomized trials may therefore become problematic. However, if individuals do consent to participate in a randomized trial, it is possible that having a preference/dislike for an intervention could enhance/reduce their response (possibly through compliance or via a psychological pathway) and the randomized trial may give misleading results.

The effects of participant preferences will be least when a randomized controlled trial is 'blinded' (that is, the recipient is unaware as to which intervention arm of the trial they have been allocated), but blinding is often impossible, particularly for health promotion initiatives. For example, it would be impossible to blind participants to whether they were receiving counselling for smoking cessation compared to hypnosis therapy. An individual may have strong beliefs in the effectiveness of hypnosis, and if randomized to this arm of the trial may experience an enhanced response, above and beyond the intervention's intrinsic effect. It is very difficult to measure the consequences of preference effects, if they exist (McPherson *et al.* 1997), but researchers need to be aware of them when planning trials.

Unique features of health promotion

The strengths and weaknesses of randomized controlled trials have important implications for the ways in which evaluative research in health promotion is conducted, interpreted, and reported. Rigorous evaluation is important, but that does not mean that a randomized controlled trial is the best method in every circumstance. The aims of health promotion differ in four important ways from those of curative interventions and these should be considered in planning or reviewing experimental studies that evaluate health promotion interventions.

Nature of the intervention

The intervention being tested in a clinical trial usually has a biological basis (for example, drugs, surgery, or physiotherapy) whereas health promotion interventions rarely involve direct manipulation of the biological environment. Health promotion interventions are aimed at achieving behavioural change at either an individual or a societal level. This has repercussions for the design of trials, both in terms of the unit which receives the intervention, (individual, community, or a whole nation), and in terms of the concepts of placebo comparisons and blinded participants. It is difficult to devise a placebo comparison intervention for a community development intervention, and almost always impossible to blind people to the fact that they have had advice or some other form of intervention aimed at changing their behaviour.

Agencies implementing the intervention

In a clinical trial, a health 'professional' will usually implement the intervention. This is true for some health promotion interventions, but many are initiated at a community level and implemented by a community body, such as a local authority, or a health promotion unit. It is relatively easy to design a trial that allocates community bodies to different intervention groups. It is much less easy to gain the cooperation of such bodies in being randomized. There is also the risk that neighbouring communities which are acting as control groups will adopt the practices of the intervention community. Such contamination is hard to prevent or control.

Nature of the clients

The recipients of health promotion interventions exist within a social context and will respond to health messages within that context. If the social context is ignored, an understanding of underlying mechanisms may be lost. Understanding the process by which an intervention operates can be as important as the final outcome.

Most health interventions in randomized controlled trials have the aim of curing or reducing a disease; in such trials participants enter with a health problem, from which they hope to find relief. In a health promotion trial, the participants are unlikely to be seeking a solution for their health problem; in fact, it is probable that the subjects do not perceive that they have a health problem. This will affect the type of people who are recruited to a trial.

Duration of effect and frequency of endpoints

One of the features of health promotion is that the interventions are intended to prevent future ill-health (physical, social, or emotional) rather than cure existing illnesses. This is equally true of community development interventions as of personalized health advice. For example, a project aimed at reducing smoking in teenage girls would have as its ultimate goals such factors as the effect on the future offspring of the girls, or the effect on lung cancer rates in the girls when they had reached late middle age. The focus of health promotion on outcomes in the (often distant) future makes it difficult to design and run suitable randomized controlled trials. Apart from the expense, and the delay in obtaining useful results, it would usually prove to be impossible to ensure that the intervention arms continued to differ in the way that had been planned. As people move areas, or join new friendship groups, and so on, the resulting contamination would rapidly dilute any effect of the intervention. As time passes, the certainty of attribution diminishes.

Implications for the evaluation of health promotion

The evaluation of health promotion interventions presents particular problems. Randomized controlled trials clearly have their place (Stephenson and Imrie 1998). For example, researchers in California wanted to find the best way to encourage increased physical activity amongst sedentary people in late middle age. They sought volunteers for the trial by random digit dialling in the local community and then randomized the subjects to one of four groups. One was a control group who were simply assessed for fitness, while the other three were given varying advice on taking exercise. Two groups were recommended to undertake home-based exercise, one of high intensity and one of low intensity, while the third group was recommended to join a high-intensity group-based exercise plan. At the end of the trial, the researchers concluded that home-based exercise was as effective as group exercise, and that low-intensity exercise (such as brisk walking) was as effective as high-intensity exercise. The results of trials such as this are important in the development of new strategies to increase activity and improve fitness (King *et al.* 1991).

However, there are limitations to randomized controlled trials and they are often impossible in health promotion. This is not an excuse for failing to evaluate health promotion. Other methods of evaluation must be sought, and the merits of alternative study designs need to be explored. The need for a sound evidence base for health promotion is as important as for other public health fields.

Alternative forms of experimental evaluation

It may prove impossible, for practical reasons, to use a randomized controlled trial to evaluate an initiative. When this is the case, other forms of experimental evaluation should be considered. These will lose something in 'internal validity' but may gain in 'external validity'. They can be considered in two categories: those where comparison groups can be identified but randomization is not possible; and those where no comparison group can be identified. In either case, developing a good quality research protocol requires careful thought, and often, some ingenuity.

Studies with a current comparison group but without randomization

The three most important considerations in such studies are, firstly, to make every effort to ensure that the study is big enough to detect the difference that one is expecting to see; secondly to find comparison groups which are as similar as possible to the intervention group, both with respect to the prevalence of potential confounding factors and with respect to likely external influences on the outcomes; and finally, to ensure that the important characteristics of the two groups are measured before the trial starts. For example, an ingenious study was carried out to evaluate the effect of adding fluoride to drinking water. A community in Cheshire, England, made the decision to add fluoride to the water supply, while there were no such plans in the neighbouring, very similar community that had low levels of fluoride in the water. A group of dental researchers saw this as an opportunity to evaluate the effect of fluoride in the water on post-eruptive teeth. They arranged for a sample of 12-year-old children from each of the two areas to be examined by a dentist in the year before fluoridation started, and then to be examined in the same way for the following four years, after the fluoridation had been introduced. Although they could not randomize the community which was to receive the fluoride, and could not prevent the children knowing which area they lived in, the researchers took pains to ensure that the study was single blinded. The children were bussed to a central location, and asked not to wear anything which identified their school, so that dentists who evaluated the number of caries in the teeth had no idea whether the children were from the intervention or the control area. The results showed that the students drinking the fluoridated water had 25% fewer caries at the end of the four years (Hardwick *et al.* 1982).

Such studies are not ideal, and should only be considered where randomized controlled trials are not possible. Many such studies have involved only a small number of communities and have provided inconclusive results. Many of the differences in comparison groups may be unknown or unmeasurable and so risk-adjustment techniques will not be sensitive enough to attribute the observed effects solely to the introduction of an intervention. Sub-group analysis, where closely matched people are selected from the intervention and control group and their outcomes compared, may fail because of small numbers in each sub-group.

Studies with no current comparison group

Sometimes it is not possible to find an appropriate comparison group. This is usually because the intervention being evaluated has extended over a whole population. In this case the best alternative may be for the intervention group to act as their own controls, so that the effect of the intervention is estimated from the observed change over the period of the intervention. This is sometimes described as a *before-and-after study*. In Thailand, in the late 1980s, a surveillance programme was set up to monitor the spread of HIV. Between 1989 and 1991 a rapid increase in the prevalence of infection in female sex workers was noted, from a 3.5% to a 15% prevalence. In response, the Ministry of Public Health set up the '100% condom campaign' to control the spread of infection. Condoms were provided to every establishment where sex was sold and their use was strongly encouraged. This was a national campaign, so no current control group was available. The initiative was evaluated by a study of a series of five cohorts of army recruits between 1991 and 1995. Between 1991 and 1993 the prevalence of HIV in army recruits ranged between 10 and 13%; by 1995, it had fallen to 7%, and in men who reported having no sexual relations with a female sex worker until after 1992 the prevalence was 0.7% (Nelson *et al.* 1996). Before-and-after studies have many weaknesses and should only be considered when other types of trial are not possible. However, as with the evaluation of the Thai 100% condom campaign, they can provide useful evidence of whether or not an intervention may be effective.

Choosing an appropriate experimental design

When conducting research, particularly within the field of health promotion evaluation, the choice of whether to use a randomized or non-randomized strategy will probably be dictated by practicalities. Figure 4.1 illustrates the basic questions to be addressed. Once a method of evaluation has been chosen, the work is only just beginning. The challenge is to design and carry out the most reliable and valid study possible. To help with the design stage, it is important to consider a number of questions, detailed in Box 4.1.

Fig. 4.1 Choosing an experimental study design in health promotion.

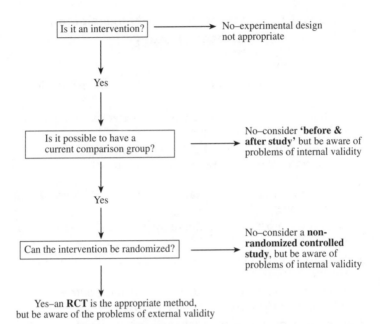

Randomized controlled trials are typically perceived as providing the most reliable and valid evidence, but their use in health promotion has been criticized (Speller *et al.* 1997). There has been criticism from some health promoters about the perceived dominance of the biomedical approach which imposes inappropriate rules and fails to take account of the long duration and complex nature of most health promotion interventions. The lack of RCT evidence should not be interpreted as a weakness of health promotion interventions. Well-conducted non-randomized studies, corroborated by other qualitative evidence, can provide a sound evidence base for health promotion interventions. Health promotion needs a strong evidence base in order to gain credibility and more importantly to ensure accuracy and effectiveness of future interventions. Because of some of the unique circumstances surrounding health promotion interventions, a number of types of study need to be used.

Box 4.1   Questions to ask when designing a research study

All study designs:

1. Is your study group representative of the wider population of interest?

2. Is your sample size large enough to detect an intervention effect? (Consult a statistician.)

3. How will you deal with people who do not comply with the study protocol or who are lost at follow up?

If a randomized controlled trial has been chosen, think about these questions:

1. What is the most efficient unit of randomization (individual or cluster)?

2. Is it possible to blind the trial participants to the allocation of the intervention and control?

3. Is it possible to blind the people measuring the outcome to the allocation of the intervention and control?

4. At what stage of the study will randomization occur?

If a non-randomized controlled trial has been chosen, think about these questions:

1. Are the intervention and control groups similar for known confounders?

2. Can known confounders be measured at baseline and adjusted for in the analysis?

If a study with no current comparison group is chosen, think about these questions:

1. Are there any identifiable time trends (apart from the planned intervention) which are likely to distort the results? Can these be measured and adjusted for?

2. Is it possible to identify a sample (of individuals or small communities) which can be studied at baseline and then at points during and after the intervention?

3. If not, how will the expected change in the population be measured?

Key points

- Randomized controlled trials, if well conducted, are a valid and important way of evaluating health promotion interventions.

- RCTs, however, are not always appropriate or possible and other forms of study, including non-randomized controlled trials and before-and-after studies can provide useful evidence.

- RCTs are useful for measuring the effects of interventions but not for explaining why these effects occur.

References

Britton, A., McKee, M., Black, N., McPherson, K., Sanderson, D., and Bain, C. (1998). Choosing between randomized and non-randomized studies. A systematic review. *Health Technology Assessment*, **2**(13), XX–XX.

Buck, C., Llopis, A., Najera, E., and Terris M. (ed.) (1988). *The challenge of epidemiology. Issues and selected readings*. Pan American Health Organisation, Washington.

Chalmers, I. and Altman, D. G. (1995). *Systematic reviews*. BMJ Publishing Group, London.

Hardwick, J. L., Teasdale, J., and Bloodworth, G. (1982). Caries increments over 4 years in children aged 12 at the start of the water fluoridation. *British Dental Journal*, **153**, 73–8.

King, A. C., Haskell, W. L., Taylor, B., Kraemer, H. C., and DeBusk RF. (1991). Group—vs home-based exercise training in healthy older men and women. *Journal of the American Medical Association*, **266**, 1535–42.

McPherson, K., Britton, A. R., and Wennberg, J. E. (1997). Are randomised controlled trials controlled? Patient preferences and unblind trials. *Journal of the Royal Society of Medicine*, **90**, 652–6.

Nelson, K. E., Celentano, D. D., Eimtrakol, S., Hoover, D. R., Beyrer, C., Suprasert, S. *et al.* (1996). Changes in sexual behaviour and a decline in HIV infection among young men in Thailand. *New England Journal of Medicine*, **335**, 297–303.

NHS Centre for Reviews and Dissemination (1996). *Undertaking systematic reviews of research on effectiveness: CRD guidelines for those carrying out or commissioning reviews*. CRD Report No 4. NHS Centre for Reviews and Dissemination, York.

Pocock S. J., (1997). *Clinical trials. A practical approach*. Wiley, Chichester.

Schultz, K. F., Chalmers, I., Hayes, R. J., and Altman, D. G. (1995). Empirical evidence of bias. Dimensions of methodological quality associated with estimates of treatment effects in controlled trials. *Journal of the American Medical Association*, **273**(5), 408–12.

Speller, V., Learmounth, A., and Harrison, D. (1997). The search for evidence of effective health promotion. *British Medical Journal*, **315**, 361–3.

Stephenson, J. and Imrie, J. (1998). Why do we need randomised controlled trials to assess behavioural interventions? *British Medical Journal*, **316**, 611–13.

5

....

The role of focus groups in evaluation

P. Branigan and K. Mitchell

A focus group is a method of group interview which explicitly includes and uses the group interaction to generate data. The essence of the focus group approach is this interaction between group members, so that attempts must be made to enable participants to focus on one another, rather than on the researcher (Kitzinger 1994). This chapter looks at the role of focus groups in evaluating health promotion interventions. The potential of focus groups for this purpose has not been fully explored. Focus groups can be a valid stand-alone evaluation technique, but they are currently most often used in combination with other qualitative and quantitative methods.

This chapter is not designed to show 'how to do it', but more to show 'what is possible'. A more practical approach to techniques can be found in other texts (Kitzinger 1995; Krueger 1994).

The growing importance of the focus group technique in social science

There has been growing interest in the use of qualitative

methods in conducting evaluations (Patton 1990; Steckler *et al.*
1992), with many evaluation practitioners now looking for
ways to integrate both qualitative and quantitative methods
(Chapter 3). Development of this group interview technique
within social sciences has trailed behind the rapid popu-
larization of the approach in market research. In the 1950s
the method was first applied to the marketing field and by
1960 was widely recognized as a legitimate tool. Today it is
viewed as one of the most important consumer research
techniques available and is pervasively used in market research.

Use of the focus group in community health research has
its grounding in the international health arena of the 1970s,
with the introduction of social marketing in family planning
(Manoff 1985). In this case it was the pharmaceutical companies providing the materials, and these companies were
already familiar with the marketing approach to promotion.
Social marketing approaches, qualitative research, and group
interviews have been slow to diffuse into the domain of
public health, largely because of the traditional quantitative
bias of biomedicine and epidemiology. Researchers who have
chosen focus groups as an evaluative technique have had to
struggle with limited resources for practical guidance, lack of
precision regarding appropriate uses of different types of
focus group, and conflicting viewpoints on the strengths
and weaknesses of these methods in health promotion
(Coreil 1995). The more recent history of focus groups in
the social sciences has been one of both considerable borrow-
ing and innovation.

Functions of focus groups in health promotion evaluation

Focus groups can allow collection of details at the design
stage to answer open-ended, in-depth questions. Health promotion interventions operate in three broad stages. The first
stage is that of planning and design, the second stage is the

implementation, and the third stage consists of observing the effects of the initiative or evaluation. Focus groups can be used in all three stages of evaluating health promotion interventions. The focus group method is versatile and can be used to:

- qualitatively evaluate programmes or specific aspects of programmes;
- develop questions for use in a questionnaire;
- review results from quantitative questionnaires to help interpret the results and provide case studies;
- develop general ideas on methods for an intervention to achieve a particular behaviour change;
- develop or refine specific procedures for components of an intervention;
- develop ideas and themes for use in mass media productions;
- evaluate early drafts (concept/storyboard stages) of mass media campaigns.

This flexible range of uses for focus groups in health promotion contrasts markedly with the marketing applications of focus groups in which they have historically served as a preliminary step to be followed by quantitative research (McQuarrie 1996).

There are three broad categories of focus group use. First, they can be used as a self-contained method in studies where they provide the principal source of data. In these cases focus groups are a stand-alone evaluation technique. Use of focus groups in this manner requires a careful matching of the goals of the research project with the data that the focus groups can produce, and the use of focus groups in this way often leads to an emphasis on research design. Focus groups as a self contained method have been used to evaluate a wide range of projects from osteoporosis services and women's health promotion services to the evaluation of the State programme component of the Australian National Better Health Program (Baum *et al.* 1996).

Second, they can be used as supplementary sources of data in studies that rely on some other primary method, such as a survey. The groups must then be set up and conducted in ways that maximize their value for the primary method. Such a use was the evaluation of quality of life questionnaire for people suffering from Irritable Bowel Syndrome.

Third, they are used in multi-method studies that combine two or more data gathering means. Methodological triangulation (using two or more methods to test the same hypothesis) can be used to enhance the reliability and validity of the data. The place of research groups in this mix of methods would depend on the researcher's data needs, and the opportunities and limitations of the setting.

The role of focus groups in formative evaluation

One reason for evaluation is to improve the design of an intervention, either prior to implementation (through pre-testing) or for future introduction of similar initiatives (by linking evaluation findings to future similar plans). Focus groups can play an important part in pre-testing, developing, and designing health promotion mass media campaign materials and messages. Pre-testing helps to ensure that tailored health promotion messages and projects are developed for particular, defined, target audiences. It is essential to explore the characteristics of the target group as well as the appropriate language, settings, and communication media of the proposed initiative.

The extent to which there is anything confusing, conflicting, or contradictory in the message or design should be explored to investigate any unintended outcomes of the intervention. A key role for focus groups is the analysis of unintended outcomes such as 'denial' strategies among target audiences, or alternatively, information that encourages undesirable behaviour. A further problem arises from non-target audience members taking offence to the message.

A common misconception about focus groups is that they are a quick, easy, and cheap method of evaluation. Focus group research can be as detailed and lengthy a process as a clinical trial. For example, the Best Start Project, which aimed to promote breast-feeding among economically disadvantaged women in the south-eastern United States of America, used focus groups in the formative evaluation of a social marketing approach (Bryant *et al.* 1992). The data were collected for this project over a period of two years and a large budget was required.

Although the principles involved in focus group techniques owe much to the specialities of marketing and advertising, focus groups can be used much more widely than merely in relation to mass media health promotion campaigns. Focus group data can inform the choice of words or phrases in a questionnaire, the construction of items to measure a given concept, the formation of new hypotheses, and the development of survey procedures.

The role of focus groups in process and outcome evaluation

The implementation and maintenance of an intervention are together referred to as the process. Process evaluation offers feedback on what took place when a particular programme or activity was implemented. It attempts to explain how certain results occurred by looking at what factors in the implementation process were instrumental and which factors were of benefit, or conversely, hindered progress towards the aims of the programme. This includes both factors internal to the work, and external factors which impacted on the work. The kind of information that might be obtained from focus groups include:

- information on the roles of the campaign participants, and dynamics between them;
- knowledge of the organizational model that underpins the activity;
- the perceived history of the initiative;
- the social and political context, particularly those features of the social context which facilitate or impede change;

- the extent to which the participants of a health promotion intervention found it a positive experience;
- the quality of specific programme components.

Focus groups can be a useful method of evaluating the relevance, clarity, and practicality of health promotion material or even clinical practice guidelines at the inception of a project or at a later revision stage. Focus groups were used in the qualitative evaluation of the Canadian Medical Association's counselling guidelines for HIV testing. The research groups provided detailed, credible, and consistent data about the face and content validity of the guidelines (Rowan *et al.* 1996). Another role is the updating and redesigning of health promotion materials that may need adjustment to maintain their relevance. Such an example is the updating of the Terrence Higgins Trust 'Time to Test' booklets where a series of focus groups were used to provide input into the style, tone, and content.

A distinction is commonly made between process and outcome evaluation. However, as Downie *et al.* (1996) suggest, there is no consistent distinguishing line between measures of process and measures of outcome. Indicators which may be measures of process in one situation may be measures of outcome in another and these indicators may be measured using focus groups.

The use of focus groups in evaluation: some important considerations

The creative and developmental nature of many health promotion strategies need to be matched by correspondingly creative and varied evaluation strategies. As the case studies above have shown, the focus group is a flexible tool which can play a variety of roles within such an integrated and pluralistic approach. It can be used to complement other methods (such as a survey or controlled trial) or can be used alone to measure one aspect of a programme/intervention. As with any method there are a number of advantages and disadvantages, which should be considered when assessing the appropriateness of the method for a given evaluation.

Constraints of the focus group methodology

Despite their apparent simplicity and accessibility as an evaluation tool, focus groups can be time consuming, fairly expensive to run, and require skill and expertise. The group discussion is the visible tip of the iceberg; the brief middle stage in a long process which begins with planning, preparation, and recruitment and ends in analysis and detailed reports. The recruitment of participants from outside a particular project, as in the formative evaluation of campaign materials, tends to be either expensive (if undertaken by a private recruitment firm) or time consuming (if undertaken by the in-house evaluation team). Rigorous analysis requires time and expertise and relies on accurate recording of discussions. Accurate recording, in turn, relies on superior recording equipment and acquired transcribing skills. That said, focus groups compare favourably with other qualitative methods in terms of time and cost; they are certainly less time consuming than participant observation and are typically faster and cheaper than individual interviews with an equivalent number of people.

There has been little quantitative evaluation of the focus group method (Sussman *et al.* 1991). Major advocates of focus groups (Kitzinger 1995; Krueger 1994) recognize that there are factors which can make it difficult to obtain the opinions and perceptions of all group members. Thus, it has been suggested that a focus group may be considered a sample of one (instead of a sample of the number of members of the group) (Morgan 1988). Reliability of estimation is also a particular problem of focus group research. The number of focus groups which would be necessary in order to reliably estimate different kinds of phenomena has not been investigated. Evaluators using focus groups should be wary of assuming that they have unbiased information after conducting just four or five groups. A similar concern is that questions may not be consistently asked across all project focus groups, resulting in the responses reflecting answers to substantially different questions. Thus, tabulation of responses from focus groups cannot be accepted as estimates of the prevalence and must also be interpreted with caution.

Another potential problem is the presence of power differentials within the focus group. This could be a differential between participants or between the participants and the moderator, evaluator, or research team. Focus groups can sometimes encounter problems within established settings, particularly when used to elicit the views of people related to each other in hierarchies. This is because, during a group discussion, the views of subordinate individuals are likely to be muted by the opinions of the dominant. Take, for example, a process evaluation of a health promotion campaign in a prison setting. A focus group which brought together junior and senior prison officers, or even prison staff and prisoners, might give rise to acquiescent responses from the subordinate members and fail to uncover the true problems and barriers. The same principle applies when bringing together the providers and recipients of a programme within the same focus group. Alternatively, the focus group may stir up pre-existing frustrations and antagonisms unrelated to the evaluation.

For the researcher, one option is to treat these difficult dynamics as data in themselves. Alternatively, separate groups may be convened for stakeholders with different perspectives/interests. Although more likely to engender honest opinions, such groups cannot provide first-hand observation of the dynamics between different groups which might impact on the implementation process. The choice will depend on a realistic assessment of staff hierarchies and dynamics, but also on the particular aims of the evaluation. It should also be borne in mind that extrovert individuals can dominate group discussions irrespective of their status. Focus groups seem to work well when participants feel a comfort and freedom to share their experiences and when participants feel that their suggestions and comments will be listened to and taken seriously.

A frequent problem is the ability of the moderator to understand the culture and language of the target audience. Krueger, a major advocate of focus groups, argues that

'The moderator should be fluent in the language of the target audience, have an in-depth understanding of the culture and then seek wisdom from local experts as he/she interprets the findings.' (R. A. Krueger, personal correspondence)

A related drawback of the focus group method is 'group think' where individuals adjust their views in response to their perception of what other members think. This process can build and establish group norms which effectively silence contradictory views held by individuals. There are various ways of minimising this bias, including the use of a devil's advocate to present the other side of the argument. This tactic can be made transparent and played by a group member who explains their role from the outset. Where an advocate role is inappropriate, a skilled moderator, able to detect 'group think' in action, may decide to throw in a contradictory remark themselves. 'Group think' is most likely to be an issue where there are established hierarchies between group members and where the topic under discussion is sensitive.

For many small-scale or tightly budgeted health promotion initiatives, in-house evaluation is the only feasible option. Sometimes this means that the individual or organization implementing the programme is also responsible for evaluating it. Objectivity is more difficult to achieve where evaluators have a vested interest in the success of the programme. Bias can creep into the wording of questions, moderator handling of negative views, and selective attention to transcript quotes. But equally, bias can come from focus group members who either want to agree with the moderator (acquiescence bias) or want to be regarded in a positive light generally (desirability bias).

A moderator neutral to the outcome of the evaluation can also encounter difficulties with acquiescence or desirability bias. He or she may find it difficult to convince participants that he/she is independent of the intervention and that negative viewpoints are as valuable as positive ones. Desirability bias can be a problem in any evaluation method and is not a good reason to avoid using focus groups since a sensitivity to and awareness of the problem can do much to minimize the impact.

Focus groups with participants who are inarticulate or have language difficulties can be challenging but not impossible. It is often precisely such people that health promotion initiatives are attempting to reach and an intervention that claims a client-centred approach has a responsibility to take account of their opinions. Given the right conditions, focus groups can often provide a 'safe' environment for the expression of views which individuals might find difficult to articulate on their own (in an interview) or on paper (in a survey). Kitzinger (1990) successfully undertook focus group research with pre-existing groups to evaluate the impact of AIDS media messages on various diverse audiences including office cleaners, young male prostitutes, and members of a retirement club.

Finally another problem associated with conducting a large number of research groups is the associated management challenge of a large amount of textual data. This becomes a test of data management, processing, analysis, and reporting skills, which is often compounded by a short research time scale.

Strengths of the focus group methodology

Perhaps the most important advantage of focus group research over other qualitative methods is the use of group interaction to generate data. Group members stimulate each other to think and express opinions, which in turn stimulates more thought. The focus group canvasses a range of views and opinions without necessarily presenting a consensus view. Group interaction can provide valuable insights and ideas, and raise questions not previously considered by programme organizers or evaluators. Ideas raised during the formative evaluation stage can be incorporated prior to the intervention. Equally, problems identified during the process evaluation may be addressed during the course of the intervention.

The focus group method is particularly useful for community development projects, which rely on participants to set the agenda and aim to be responsive to changing and ongoing needs. Used in this context, the focus group can be an empowering approach to evaluation enabling participants to 'own' the evaluation process to some degree.

Focus groups can answer pertinent questions about an intervention such as: Is it ethical? Why did some participants drop out? What aspects of the intervention did participants find particularly beneficial? Focus groups can also explore relevant cultural and political factors and identify organizational barriers to successful implementation. Unintended outcomes of interventions can often come to light during focus group discussions. Their particular strength lies in gathering general views, assessing priorities, and understanding cultural beliefs. They are less good at exploring personal experiences and sensitive issues, although this depends to an extent on the skill of the moderator.

Focus groups with established natural groups can provide invaluable insights to process evaluation. Focus group researchers are increasingly entertaining the idea that non-researchers, such as individuals involved in implementing an intervention, can provide a unique contribution to the research by providing insight and understanding of the project that a researcher from outside does not possess.

The future role for focus groups in evaluation

Recent development of qualitative software programmes (such as NUD*IST or Atlas.ti) have contributed towards a systematic approach to analysis and encouraged analysis adapted to meet specific needs. The use of focus groups in formative evaluation of mass media interventions often requires a quick turn-around, and the continuing development of analysis methodologies which can meet these timelines whilst maintaining academic rigour will become increasingly important in the future.

Focus groups are being used for evaluation by a growing number of health professionals and academics. Adequate training will be important to ensure reliable research. Researchers will continue to modify and adapt focus group interviews. The changes will be driven by emerging opportunities, technology, resources, changes in thinking, and the desire for more descriptive information (Krueger 1994). Sharing of expertise and continuing debate will be important for the future development of the methodology in health promotion evaluation.

Conclusions

Focus group research continues to gain credibility within academic and applied research. With increasing use comes the attendant potential for misuse. The inappropriate use of the focus group method not only gives rise to unreliable results but earns the method a poor reputation. If focus groups are to retain their reputation as a reliable and valid method for evaluation then there must be thorough planning, skilled moderation, and rigorous analysis. It is important to consider whether focus groups are an appropriate way to meet the aims of a project. Useful questions include: What questions can a focus group answer and how will the results be used? How will the focus group results relate to the rest of the evaluation? After these questions come practical decisions about the number and composition of groups. At this stage, time and resource constraints will become additional considerations.

Key points

- Focus groups can help in the formative stages of a health promotion campaign in identifying need, setting objectives, and pre-testing campaign materials.

- Process indicators can be tracked using focus groups.

- Focus groups can be used to measure outcome indicators of initiatives.

- They can be used effectively alongside quantitative techniques in evaluating campaigns.

- There are important considerations to the use of the focus group research tool.

References

Baum, F., Santich, B., Craig, B., and Murray, C. (1996). Evaluation of a national health programme in South Australia. *Australian and New Zealand Journal of Public Health*, **20**(1), 41–9.

Bryant, C., Coreil, J., D'Angelo, S. L., Bailey, D. F. C., and Lazarov, M. (1992). A strategy for promoting breastfeeding among economically disadvantaged women and adolescents. *NAACOG Clinical Issues in Perinatal and Women's Health Nursing*, **3**(4), 723–9.

Coreil, J. (1995). Group interview methods in community health research. *Medical Anthropology*, **16**, 193–210.

Downie, R. S., Tannahill, C., and Tannahill, A. (1996). *Health promotion: models and values* (2nd edition). Oxford University Press.

Kitzinger, J. (1990). Audience understandings of AIDS media messages: a discussion of methods. *Sociology of Health and Illness*, **12**(3), 319–35.

Kitzinger, J. (1994). The methodology of focus groups: the importance of interaction between research participants. *Sociology of Health and Illness*, **16**(1), 103–21.

Kitzinger, J. (1995). Introducing focus groups. *British Medical Journal*, **311**, 299–302.

Krueger, R. A. (1994). *Focus groups: A practical guide for applied research*. Sage, Newbury Park, California.

McQuarrie, E. F. (1996). *The market research toolbox: a concise guide for beginners*. Sage, Thousand Oaks, CA.

Manoff, R. (1985). *Social marketing: new imperative for public health*. Praeger, New York.

Morgan, D. (1988). *Focus groups as qualitative research*. Sage, Newbury Park, California.

Patton, M. (1990). *Qualitative evaluation and research methods*. Sage, Newbury Park, California.

Rowan, M. S., Toombs, M., Bally, G., Walters, D.J., and Henderson, J. (1996). Qualitative evaluation of the Canadian Medical Associations's counselling guidelines for HIV serologic testing. *Canadian Medical Association Journal*, **154**(5), 665–71.

Steckler, A., McLeroy, K. R., Goodman, R. M., Bird, S. T., and McCormick, L. (1992). Towards integrating qualitative and quantitative methods: an introduction. *Health Education Quarterly*, **19**(1), 1–8.

Sussman, S., Barton, D., Dent, C. W., and Stacey, A. W. (1991). Use of focus groups in developing an adolescent tobacco use cessation programme: collective norm effects. *Journal of Applied Social Psychology*, **21**, 1772–82.

6

Economic evaluation of health promotion programmes

David Wonderling and Jonathan Karnon

Although NHS resources will increase over the next few years, they will remain limited. Resources are constrained in every health service around the world. Consequently, some beneficial programmes are carried out and others are not. Economic evaluation is a tool that can help decision-makers find out which health care programmes are the best value for money. Health promotion interventions must be shown to be cost-effective if they are to compete successfully for resources.

This chapter begins by briefly explaining the general methods of economic evaluation, followed by an overview of recently published economic evaluations in one area of health promotion: smoking cessation. The methodological issues encountered in economic evaluations of health promotion programmes are then examined. Finally, the relevance of economic evaluation for health promotion is discussed.

What is economic evaluation?

Economics is concerned with choosing what to do with scarce resources. All resources (people, machinery, materials, etc.)

are considered scarce because there are not enough of them to meet all human wants. The subdiscipline of health economics is concerned with the allocation of resources within the health sector.

There is an economic cost involved every time a resource is used. This cost is equal to the benefit that would have been gained from the best alternative use of that resource. Economists describe this as an 'opportunity cost'. An allocation of resources where opportunity costs are minimized (that is, where the benefits sacrificed are smallest) is described as being efficient. Efficiency is one of the primary objectives of economics.

In the health sector, efficiency means maximizing health outcomes with a given amount of resources. It can also mean achieving a particular level of health outcome with the least amount of resources (at least cost). Suppose there are two health promotion programmes. Programme A empowers ten people to quit smoking at a cost of £1000 and Programme B has an identical impact on quitting but costs twice as much. Other things being equal, Programme A is clearly better value because the same health outcome can be achieved with fewer resources. Economists would argue that it is unethical to carry out Programme B, instead of Programme A, because there would be fewer resources left over for use in other worthwhile health programmes.

Economic evaluation is defined as 'the comparative analysis of alternative courses of action in terms of both their costs and their consequences' (Blumenschein and Johannesson 1996). It is a tool to help decision-makers allocate resources efficiently. There are essentially three different types of economic evaluation for health programmes. Each type measures health outcome in a different way and each relates to a slightly different policy problem.

Cost-effectiveness analysis (CEA)

If the cheapest way of achieving a particular health outcome is required then the most relevant health outcome is chosen. So when comparing two anti-smoking campaigns the relevant outcome might be number of smokers quitting. The preferred programme is the one with the lowest cost per quit smoker. A CEA comparison that was more broad-ranging might compare the cost per life-year gained of each programme.

Cost-utility analysis (CUA)

If the comparison is between programmes with very different outcomes then the outcome measure should incorporate both improvements in life expectancy and improvements in quality of life. One such measure is the Quality Adjusted Life Year (QALY). Weights from 0 to 1 are given to different health states according to valuations elicited from a sample population. QALYs are then equal to the length of time in a health state multiplied by the mean weight. Preferred programmes will have the lowest cost per QALY gained.

Cost-benefit analysis (CBA)

If the comparison is between a health programme and a non-health programme then CBA is more appropriate. In CBA health outcomes, as well as resources used, are valued in monetary terms. To put a monetary value on health requires asking people (or inferring from their decisions) how much they value extra years of life. The advantage of CBA is that it gives a direct answer to the question: 'Do the costs of implementing the new programme outweigh the benefits?'

The practical difficulties involved with valuing health outcomes (either with an index or in monetary terms) has meant that most economic evaluations use cost-effectiveness analysis.

Unless one programme is both less costly and more beneficial, the results of economic evaluations based on CEA or CUA are presented as cost-effectiveness ratios (for example cost per life-year gained). Cost-effectiveness league tables are sometimes produced to show which programmes are most cost-effective. Such tables are fraught with interpretational difficulties but they do provide a basis for comparison between health care programmes.

Another important economic objective is equity. Economists are concerned not only with the total impact on population health, but also with the distribution of health. Programmes that have only a moderate impact on population health but target deprived communities may be considered as important as a programme that has a larger impact on population health. Consequently, while efficiency is an important criterion, it can only inform, and not replace, decision-making.

Case-study: smoking cessation programmes

Within the past few years, economic evaluations of individual counselling, group therapy, and replacement therapies (nicotine patches or gum), have been published (see Table 6.1). Such interventions have been undertaken in a range of locations including GP surgeries, hospitals, nicotine dependence centres, and military medical centres. Cost-effectiveness studies have also been undertaken for mass media campaigns.

Table 6.1 uses recent economic evaluations of smoking cessation programmes to illustrate the variety of methodological approaches taken in this one area of evaluation. It also shows the general convergence of the reported cost-effectiveness of such programmes—certainly at the lower ends of the reported ranges these programmes appear to be very good value for money. However, the different types of outcomes measured and other methodological differences restrict cross-study comparisons.

Methodological issues

1. Comparators

Within any evaluation, economic or otherwise, the choice of comparator(s) is crucial; the comparison intervention(s) should be the most relevant for the policy question being addressed. In many health care areas, the relevant comparator will be the most commonly used existing therapy. However,

Table 6.1 Recent economic evaluations of smoking cessation interventions

Reference & origin	Alternatives compared	Outcomes reported	Costs included	Discount rate	Year of analysis	Results
Cromwell et al. (1997); USA	5 counselling interventions (minimal, brief, full, individual intensive and group intensive) with or without nicotine replacement (transdermal nicotine and nicotine gum)	life years saved, QALYs saved	programme costs and costs of gum, and patches to participants	3% for outcomes	1995	$2186–488962 per quitter, $1496–$6135 per life year saved
Fiscella and Franks (1996); USA	counselling, counselling + nicotine patch	QALYs saved	costs of patch and extra physician time in offering the patch**	3%	1995	men; $4390–10943 and women; $4995–6983 per QALY gained
Goldman and Glantz (1998); USA	two separate advertising campaigns	fall in number of packs of cigarettes per capita per year per capita dollar	programme costs to State	N/A*	1996	0.5–3.9 packs per capita per year per capita dollar
Meenan et al. (1998); USA	programme for hospitalized smokers	life years gained	programme costs	5% for outcomes	1994	$94–7444 per life year gained
Mudde et al. (1996); Holland	advertising campaign and phone line leading to self help manual vs group programme	quitters	programme costs, and time and travel costs to participants, presented separately and together	N/A*	1990	$37–1412 per quitter
Ratcliffe et al. (1997); Scotland	advertising campaign and phone line leading to self help manual vs group programme	quitters, life years saved	campaign costs	0% and 6% for outcomes	1992/3	£168–369 per quitter, £92–656 per life year saved
Warner et al. (1996); USA	workplace programme	cessation, death postponed, life years saved	programme costs to employer, savings in health cars costs, absenteeism costs, productivity and health insurance	3.5% for costs and outcomes	1995	$1029–1500 per cessation, $21449–372875 per death postponed, $894–99703 per life year saved

* N/A: not applicable

** Costs attributable to both programmes were not included, therefore, unable to compare to a baseline rate of quitting.

many smoking cessation interventions are not continuously employed, and the wealth of possible alternatives makes the choice of comparator difficult. Published studies, which have included an active comparator, have tended to pick comparators of a similar ilk to the intervention of interest, such as comparing the use of nicotine patches and counselling with counselling alone (Fiscella and Franks 1996). As more economic evaluations of smoking cessation interventions are undertaken, a clearer idea of which interventions are most cost effective will be established. Given the lack of commonly used existing therapies, such interventions may be the most appropriate comparators. To enable comparison with alternative interventions in other studies it would be helpful if every evaluation had a do-nothing comparator (that is, the natural rate of smoking cessation) so that a common baseline exists.

2. Mode of evaluation

The data used in an economic evaluation can come from an intervention study (see Chapter 4), an observational study, or a modelling exercise (see Chapter 8). Of course, like any quantitative study it should be informed and complemented by qualitative studies (see Chapter 3).

An advantage of using clinical trials is that patient-specific data can be collected for both costs and outcomes, which is helpful for analysis, and boosts internal validity. Although clinical trials are regarded as the gold standard for establishing efficacy, the associated controlled conditions generate particular problems for generalizability. Observational studies may provide more naturalistic data, and allow a larger sample to be followed, although internal validity will be compromised (see Chapter 4).

Empirical studies are rarely designed with economic evaluation at the forefront, therefore problems sometimes arise with respect to the choice of comparators, sample size and follow-up. Models may be used to synthesize cost and outcome data from various sources in cases where specific empirical work is inadequate or where the intermediate outcomes need extrapolating to provide useful economic endpoints. Modelling can be especially useful if the relevant alternatives focus on different populations, for example an individual-based smoking cessation programme and a mass media campaign.

Simulation models (Chapter 8) have been used for the economic evaluation of smoking cessation interventions (Ratcliffe *et al.* 1997; Warner *et al.* 1996). As smoking cessation programmes persuade smokers to quit, the remaining core of smokers are those who will find it most difficult to give up. Therefore the cost-effectiveness of smoking cessation interventions will change over time. Simulation models can incorporate this effect. Indeed simulations can be used to test a whole range of assumptions. While there are a number of computer models that can be used to estimate the changes in mortality (and changes in costs) corresponding to changes in particular risk factors, morbidity is harder to model.

3. *Cost measurement*

Costs are the value (or price) of the resources used. Resources include the time of professionals and workers, consumables (syringes, leaflets, etc.), and the use of buildings and equipment. The study perspective and time frame adopted determine which costs should be included.

Study perspective

In addition to the direct costs of a health promotion programme there may be cost implications for the subjects and their families. For example, the participants in a programme that encourages people to exercise might incur the costs of gym fees and sports equipment. Although the measurement of such costs adds to the work of the researcher, it does not create any major difficulty.

As well as having resource implications for participants and families, a health promotion programme may have resource implications for other health and social services. Sometimes the consequence will be increased costs for the health service and sometimes cost savings.

The inclusion of the different costs types (programme costs, patient costs, health service costs, etc.) is primarily guided by the perspective taken for an evaluation. In general, economic evaluations are conducted from a health service or societal perspective; both these perspectives have been adopted in the smoking cessation literature.

Cromwell *et al.* (1997) identified four main categories of direct programme costs for an individual based intervention:
- screening the population for smokers;
- advising smokers;
- motivating smokers to quit; and
- the employment of non-smoking aids.

Mudde *et al.* (1996) also included the time and travel costs to patients of attending group programmes. An unusual perspective, almost unique to health promotion, is that of the employer. Several studies of smoking cessation interventions have taken this perspective; for example, Warner *et al.* (1996) included programme planning, recruiting participants, securing space, etc. In addition, cost savings for the firm included reductions in health care costs, absenteeism costs, on-the-job productivity costs, and life insurance costs.

Study time frame

Health promotion programmes may impact on future resource use. If a health promotion programme results in people living healthy lives then, in the medium term, health service costs are reduced because fewer people will be contracting diseases. But in the long term there may be no cost savings because people are living longer and consuming additional health services. The extent to which long term costs are included varies markedly between studies.

The time frame of an evaluation will influence the resulting costs greatly. Many published evaluations have restricted cost collection to the direct costs of providing the intervention. However, excluding the future financial implications of smoking cessation interventions may hide important cost considerations. In the examples for smoking cessation above, only Warner *et al.* (1996) measured future health care cost savings.

It is generally accepted that health care costs falling outside the condition of interest should not be included, although there is still some debate. Applying this logic to smoking cessation programmes means that the measurement of future health care costs should consider all costs associated with illnesses attributable to smoking. Such costs can only be incorporated into an evaluation using data synthesized from different sources. Plenty of work has been completed separately on the lifetime costs of smokers and non-smokers (see for example Barendregt *et al.* 1997), however, the assumptions should be carefully scrutinized.

4. Measurement of outcomes

The most common outcome measures in economic evaluations of smoking cessation interventions include the number of quitters, life years saved, and quality adjusted life years (QALYs) saved. The choice of outcome is important with respect to the objective of the evaluation. For example, an evaluation reporting the cost per quitter could not be used to compare the relative cost-effectiveness of a smoking cessation intervention with a kidney transplant programme. Conversely, the effort involved in calculating the cost per QALY might be ill spent if the objective was to fund the most cost-effective smoking cessation intervention.

If comparisons are between very different interventions then health outcome needs to be measured broadly. The health effects of a health promotion programme may be very broad, impacting on several different health risks. An intervention with a goal of reducing coronary heart disease through lifestyle advice may have additional health improvements such as reduced lung cancer and stroke.

Many outcomes of health promotion programmes occur in the long term and are difficult and costly to measure. However, there are usually some intermediate outcomes which can be measured, such as changes in risk factors. In the case of smoking cessation, the health effects can be modelled from patient characteristics at the time of smoking cessation. Ratcliffe *et al.* (1997) used the Prevent model (see Chapter 8) to extrapolate the life years gained from the estimated quit rate. Other studies have used age-specific mortality rates for smokers and non-smokers to calculate differences in life years gained (Cromwell *et al.* 1997; Fiscella and Franks 1996; Meenan *et al.* 1998). Cromwell *et al.* (1997) and Fiscella and Franks (1996) applied quality adjustments using published weights to calculate QALYs gained.

5. Discounting

Discounting is the adjustment of future costs and benefits to their present value. There are a number of reasons for putting a lower weight on costs and benefits in the future. One reason is that money available in the present can be invested to earn interest and therefore accumulate value; thus, a pound today is valued higher than a pound available in one year's time. To account for this time preference health care expenditures occurring in the future are discounted.

Unfortunately, there is no consensus regarding the discounting of health effects, as time preference for such effects has not been definitively revealed. Among the studies presented in Table 6.1, the yearly discount rate applied to health outcomes ranged from 0% to 6%.

It is sometimes claimed that discounting health benefits disadvantages health promotion activities because the benefits often occur in the distant future. This is true to some extent, however, any programme which affects mortality will be similarly disadvantaged compared with programmes that yield immediate improvements in quality of life. It is important that all economic evaluations test the sensitivity of the results to the discount rate assumed.

6. Spillover of interventions

A health promotion programme may be transferred to other members of the community. A campaign that informs people about the benefits of healthy eating might have a wider impact than just on the original target group. Targeted individuals pass on the information to friends and relatives outside of the intervention. These spillover effects can be estimated although it may be difficult to identify precisely the number of people indirectly affected by the intervention.

The effects of smoking cessation interventions may have been underestimated if it is the case that helping some individuals to stop smoking removes peer pressure for other smokers, thus encouraging smoking cessation outside of the interventions.

7. Programme scale

The cost-effectiveness of some health promotion activities will vary greatly according to the scale of the programme. For example, the costs of a mass media campaign will rise less than proportionally as the campaign is spread over a larger geographical area. This is because some of the design and production costs are only incurred once regardless of the population covered. In this case, the researcher could calculate the minimum population size required to make the campaign cost-effective. For more general discussions of the methodological issues see Drummond *et al.* (1997) and Gold *et al.* (1996).

How useful are economic evaluations for health promotion?

In every country the resources available for health care and public health programmes are limited. It is therefore important (and ethical) that programmes adopted are those with a large impact on population health relative to the resources they consume. Economic evaluation is useful because it allows decision-makers to compare the relative value for money of different health care programmes.

There are certain characteristics of health promotion programmes that make measuring their costs and benefits problematic (as described in the section above). Burrows *et al.* (1995) have argued that economic evaluation cannot and should not be applied to health promotion at all. They argue that most health promotion research is not based on experimental study. This certainly does not need to be the case (see Chapter 4). They also argue that causal relationships cannot be drawn out for behavioural studies in the same way that they can for biomedical interventions. Craig and Walker (1996) argue that this is overstated, for there are a number of health promotion activities with almost irrefutable evidence of effectiveness. They add that chains of arguments can be used to analyse final health impacts. For example, the impact of smoking on health is well documented, therefore evaluations of smoking cessation programmes can focus on quit rates. Thus evaluation techniques can be, and are, tailored to answer particular policy questions. The practical difficulties are reduced if the policy question is more focused.

Burrows *et al.* (1995) also argue that economic techniques do not provide objective measures of overall benefit. For example, broad measures of health outcome, such as QALYs, inevitably involve value judgements about the relative importance of different health effects. Craig and Walker (1996) point out that health economists would agree with these statements. The value of the economic approach is that an attempt is made to systematically evaluate all the consequences of a programme. A trade-off of different costs and benefits is implicitly made in any resource allocation decision. Economic evaluation brings the trade-off into the open with all assumptions made explicit. Because such trade-offs inevitably involve value judgements, economic evaluation can only inform decision-making and cannot replace it.

That Burrows and colleagues could have misunderstood the claims of economic evaluation is not surprising. Health economists and health care decision-makers do sometimes overstate the importance of efficiency. Tolley *et al.* (1996) advocate three desirable objectives:

- Economists should not shy away from evaluating health promotion programmes and they should further develop evaluative techniques.
- Health promotion researchers should be taught the usefulness of the health economic framework.
- Decision-makers should be educated so that they do not blindly use narrow economic evaluations that appear to favour treatment interventions.

These objectives can only be achieved by increasing dialogue between health promotion specialists, health economists and health decision-makers.

Although evaluating health promotion involves some practical difficulties, the process is not fundamentally different to any other health economic evaluation. Furthermore, the existence of scarcity and rationing in the health sector means that there is a moral imperative to estimate the relative value for money of health promotion programmes.

Key points

- Economics is relevant in health promotion as it is in health care generally because the resources that are available cannot meet all effective health promoting activities.

- Economic evaluation seeks to measure the costs (resources used) and overall health benefits of health promoting activities.

- Health promotion programmes create complications for economic evaluation, not least because they have diverse and long-lasting consequences for health and resource use.

- Economic evaluations have been successfully carried out for a number of health promotion programmes.

- It is important that economic evaluations are designed around relevant policy questions and that the methods employed are chosen carefully.

References

Barendregt, J. J., Bonneux, L., and van der Maas, P. J. (1997). The health care costs of smoking. *New England Journal of Medicine*, **337**, 1052–7.

Blumenschein, K. and Johannesson, M. (1996). Economic evaluation in healthcare. *Pharmacoeconomics*, **10**, 114–22.

Burrows, R., Bunton, R., Muncer, S., and Gillen, K. (1995). The efficacy of health promotion, health economics and late modernism. *Health Education Research*, **10**, 241–9.

Craig, N. and Walker, D. (1996). Choice and accountability in health promotion: the role of health economics. *Health Education Research*, **11**, 355–60.

Cromwell, J., Bartosch, W. J., Fiore, M. C., Hasselblad, V., and Baker, T. (1997). Cost-effectiveness of the clinical practice recommendations in the AHCPR guideline for smoking cessation. Agency for health care policy and research. *Journal of the American Medical Association*, **278**, 1759–66.

Drummond, M. F., O'Brien, B., Stoddart, G. L., Torrance, G. W. (1997). *Methods for the economic evaluation of health care programmes* (2nd edn). Oxford University Press.

Fiscella, K. and Franks, P. (1996). Cost-effectiveness of the transdermal nicotine patch as an adjunct to physicians' smoking cessation counseling. *Journal of the American Medical Association*, **275**, 1247–51.

Gold, M., Siegal, J., Russell, L., and Weinstein, M. (1996). *Cost-effectiveness in health and medicine*. Oxford University Press, New York.

Goldman, L. K. and Glantz, S. A. (1998). Evaluation of antismoking advertising campaigns. *Journal of the American Medical Association*, **279**, 772–7.

Meenan, R. T., Stevens, V. J., Hornbrook, M. C., La Chance, P. A., Glasgow, R. E., Hollis, J. F., *et al.* (1998). Cost-effectiveness of a hospital-based smoking cessation intervention. *Medical Care*, **36**, 670–8.

Mudde, A. N., de Vries, H., and Strecher, V. J. (1996). Cost-effectiveness of smoking cessation modalities: comparing apples with oranges? *Preventive Medicine*, **25**, 708–16.

Ratcliffe, J., Cairns, J., and Platt, S. (1997). Cost effectiveness of a mass media-led anti-smoking campaign in Scotland. *Tobacco Control*, **6**, 104–10.

Tolley, K., Buck, D., and Godfrey, C. (1996). Health promotion and health economics (Response). *Health Education Research*, **11**, 361–4.

Warner, K. E., Smith, R. J., Smith, D. G., and Fries, B. E. (1996). Health and economic implications of a work-site smoking-cessation program: a simulation analysis. *Journal of Occupational and Environmental Medicine*, **38**, 981–92.

7

....

Use of process evaluation during project implementation: experience from the CHAPS project for gay men

William Stewart

The evaluation of health promotion programmes is essential to demonstrate what constitutes effective means of providing health promotion work, and to provide data to be used in planning and implementing future health promotion work. This chapter explores some of the issues surrounding the use of process evaluation *during* the implementation of a health promotion project, using qualitative data collected as part of a process evaluation of the CHAPS (Community HIV/AIDS Prevention Strategy) programme for gay men's HIV prevention in England. This programme is funded by the UK Department of Health and led by the Terrence Higgins Trust. The chapter will illustrate some of the lessons learnt during the course of this evaluation, to provide a model for the way in which process evaluation during project implementation can best be used.

Process evaluation

A process evaluation will examine what happened when a programme was implemented, in order to examine *how* or *why*

Box 7.1 Process evaluation

Process evaluation describes what happens when a project is implemented. It can look at the direct activities in conducting a project, relations with clients or key partners, or the wider environment in which project work takes place. In doing so it can employ a number of research methods, and call on different disciplines. It aims to provide an explanation of how or why intended outcomes of the project were (or were not) brought about.

---

health promotion interventions worked or did not work. Process evaluation aims to draw links between what happened during project work and the effects of that work in order to explain the outcomes and impact. In doing so, it can identify aspects in the project implementation that contributed to specific outcomes, and avoid errors whereby good (or bad) outcomes are attributed solely to the project design rather than events during implementation.

The proper focus of a process evaluation can be construed to include three broad areas of project activity. At the centre are the actual activities of programme implementation including the design and management of the project, the functioning of the project unit, the production of resources or other services, and the activities conducted by project workers which allow contacts to take place with clients. A second area is that of the contacts between the health promotion project and the targets or clients of the project (that is, for the provision of information, counselling, or other services). Here an evaluator will also examine relations with key partners who would be expected to use or promote the services developed. Finally, an evaluator might look at the context in which a health promotion activity takes place to identify factors in the environment which were of benefit, or which hindered, progress towards its aims and objectives. This might include organizational, socio-political or economic factors which impact on project work.

The range in focus means that a wide range of qualitative

and quantitative research methods need to be employed. Programme managers may require quantitative data to allow comparison with other work. A range of quantitative measures including coverage indicators (number of people reached by a campaign), content and readability analysis of materials produced, client and provider surveys, and indicators of the quality of service by observation or by expert panel review have all been used in evaluation work (Windsor *et al.* 1994). Qualitative methods used in process evaluation include focus group discussions, unstructured or semi-structured interviews, and other ethnographic techniques such as participant observation and documentary and textual analysis.

These methods can be used in a very targeted way, to assess whether performance standards have been met, or whether the contents of a piece of health education information is comprehensible and meaningful to its target audience. Alternatively, approaches may be taken to provide a more holistic explanation of the way in which a project unfolded and was encountered by the people involved in it. This method of evaluation is described by Peter Aggleton (Aggleton and Moody 1992, p. 16) as an *illuminative* approach, which:

'tries to identify how the various elements of a health education programme were perceived and understood by those involved. It thereby aims to interpret and illuminate how and why particular outcomes were brought about. Ethnographic research methods are the ones most often used in order to do this.'

This approach, which draws from ethnography and history, argues that the contacts between workers in a project and the clients of that project are rarely straightforward since individuals may have divergent understandings of what the work is for. Therefore an approach is required which can map out and describe these divergent understandings and the way in which they impact on project work. The prolonged contact with the workers and recipients of health promotion campaigns which is needed, as well as the contextual and environmental concerns, make qualitative social research methods particularly suitable for this kind of evaluation.

In planning evaluation, a project cycle approach is often taken whereby evaluation results are only collected and used in project planning between cycles. This rigidity is often the result of the planning tools required for funders or commissioners, which specify numbers and kinds of outputs that are then difficult to change during the course of the project. This approach risks losing opportunities to improve the health promotion work being done. Project implementation is often a lengthy process, and evaluation results can be used during this process to make changes to the implementation to fine tune the approaches used, and to concentrate on methods which are proven effective, whilst discarding elements of the programme which work less well. These two approaches are compared in Fig. 7.1.

The CHAPS evaluation

Background to the CHAPS project

The examples in this chapter are taken from the evaluation of the CHAPS programme for HIV prevention among gay men in England. The CHAPS programme brought together voluntary agencies in the six cities across England chosen as having the highest prevalence of AIDS among gay men. It is led by the Terrence Higgins Trust, England's largest AIDS service organization.

In placing responsibility for gay men's health promotion work with the voluntary sector, the CHAPS project marked a new departure in the history of gay men's HIV prevention in the UK. For much of the late 1980s and early 1990s the amount of statutory funding devoted to HIV prevention among gay men was disproportionately small, given the size of the epidemic in this group (King *et al.* 1992). Despite an improvement in this situation in the early 1990s with a number of local authorities employing AIDS liaison officers for gay communities, by the time of the inception of CHAPS the epidemiological data on new HIV infections in gay men

Fig. 7.1a Fixed project design.

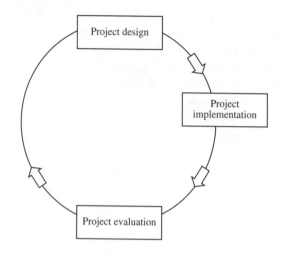

Fig. 7.1b The use of process evaluation during project implementation.

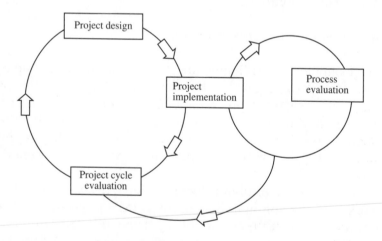

indicated that an impasse had been reached. The yearly incidence of new HIV infection was not significantly decreasing, nor was the prevalence of unprotected anal intercourse (Hickson *et al.*, unpublished review, 1985). In the early interviews for the CHAPS evaluation a recurrent theme was that more radical approaches needed to be considered as a way of 'breaking through' this static situation.

'We've still got 1500 new infections happening every year, and ...
we've been banging our heads against this wall for how long now?
And what we've got to do, we've got to do it differently.' (HIV
Prevention agency worker, CHAPS process evaluation, 1997)'

The approach taken by CHAPS was to move away from
health promotion work performed by statutory agencies, with
the restrictions placed on them, and to use voluntary organizations which are freer in the kinds of campaigns they could
produce, and were assumed to have a better understanding of
gay men's social networks.

In its design, the CHAPS programme contained both rigid
and more flexible elements. One the one hand, a series of
outputs in terms of mass media health education initiatives
was included in the project contract, which form a bulk of the
work for which CHAPS is known. In addition, a research
programme of formative and evaluation work was also commissioned. Again some elements were specified from the outset, such as a series of research briefing papers. However, the
project work undertaken by the partner agencies aside from
the Terrence Higgins Trust had a greater degree of flexibility,
being negotiated annually with the Terrence Higgins Trust,
which managed these contractual relations.

The evaluation of CHAPS

The evaluation work began in January 1997. It was felt that a
process evaluation which used the illuminative and historical
approaches outlined above was particularly suitable for a
project of this nature. There were four reasons for this. Firstly,
CHAPS sought to be an articulation or coordination of a
number of different agencies, and thus the way in which it
functions and its ultimate success would depend on relations
between these partners as they developed over the course of
the project. Research approaches were needed which could
describe these relations in order to link them to outcomes.
Secondly, the majority of these agencies pre-dated CHAPS and
were already in place with established objectives, ways of

working, funding bases, patterns of alliance, and histories vis à vis other CHAPS agencies before they became involved. An evaluative approach which was able to focus on this background was essential to understanding the processes of CHAPS as they emerged. Thirdly, as described above, CHAPS is a long term programme with a certain degree of flexibility built in. A responsive and ongoing reflexivity would also provide information on successful or less successful features of work to guide later decision-making processes. Finally, there is a difficulty of evaluating more distal, but crucial, outcomes such as sexual behaviour change, incidence of unprotected anal intercourse, and ultimately HIV infections in the case of a project such as CHAPS where there are many other interventions happening within the same communities at the same time to which these changes could be attributed. In addition, there are difficulties associated with behaviours which are also crucially affected by other sources of information outside formal health promotion initiatives. Under such circumstances it is difficult to disentangle the effects of the CHAPS work from that of other work conducted. For this reason, it was felt to be necessary to attempt to articulate the whole series of CHAPS work—from inputs and processes through to outputs in order to have any explanatory power of what the impact has or has likely been. An illuminative approach seeks to be able to make these links.

Three main fieldwork methods were used in the process evaluation, all drawn from social research.

1. *Document review*: CHAPS documents including publications within the partnership, reports of partnership meetings and weekends, campaigns materials, documents. and other occasional reports or communications were collected and reviewed.

2. *Observation*: Members of the evaluation team were present at all major meetings of the CHAPS partnership. More intense observations of case studies of specific local projects were also done.

3. *Semi-structured interviews*: Three rounds of interviews were conducted between February 1997 and March 1998. On

each round of the evaluation, semi-structured interviews were conducted face to face or by telephone with at least one representative of each partner agency using a standard interview guide. For the case studies of local working, interviews were also held with clients of health promotion projects.

To show how process evaluation can be used, and some of the difficulties encountered in its application to the CHAPS evaluation, three issues are discussed: negotiating the terms of the evaluation; the problems of shifting objectives; and evaluation of changing structures.

Negotiating the terms of an evaluation

In an evaluation employing the illuminative approach and using social research methods, prolonged contact with project workers is called for. Therefore, a process of 'negotiation' is imperative in order to allow these workers to be comfortable in giving information or opinions to evaluators. This is an essential component since, as Prout and Deverell (1995) point out, the enthusiasm for evaluation among the commissioners of health promotion work may be met by an equal amount of scepticism and concern amongst those who may feel their work is being held up to scrutiny, and it is often crucial to establish the 'independence' of the evaluation work to overcome initial antipathy.

In the evaluation of the CHAPS project this kind of a negotiation was important. Explanation of the evaluation, and of the fact that it was 'neutral' in terms of any of the organizations forming the CHAPS partnership, was required. Our intention was to offer the partners in the programme a forum where they could represent their feelings about the project as it developed, in a way which they might find difficult to do at meetings. In addition, the position of the evaluators vis à vis the other partners in CHAPS was called into question in two aspects. Firstly, in the application of research methods, a potential conflict was identified between our inclination for 'pure' observation (for example at meetings) and the trust which we found was more forthcoming

when, at meetings or partnership weekends, we also partici-
pated in discussions and offered something personal from
ourselves. Initial use of a more detached observation style
was remarked on negatively by some of the partners and a
participatory approach was adopted through which we were
able to indicate that we considered ourselves part of the
CHAPS project and not external to it, and in response we
received greater trust and more detailed data from interviews.

The second area where negotiation was necessary was in the
development of forms of feedback of research findings to the
partnership. In evaluation work, the form in which results are
fed back to the people who are intended to use the results can
be crucial in determining whether the results are seen as
constructive, and whether ultimately they are used in project
planning. In the CHAPS programme there was initially no
feedback mechanism. As evaluators, we wanted our results to
be seen as contributing to the partnership as a whole and not
just being provided for the Department of Health or the
Terrence Higgins Trust in a way which may have made workers in other agencies feel that their work was being monitored.
Through discussions with each of the partners, it was decided
that the most appropriate feedback would be through reports
and oral presentations given at the weekend retreats at which
all partners were represented.

The problem of shifting objectives

The second problem with the CHAPS evaluation, where the
illuminative approach was useful, was in tracking the shifting
nature of the objectives of CHAPS. In order to evaluate something we need to know what that thing is and what its
objectives are. We cannot judge whether something did what
it was intended to do without clarity about what was intended.
However, CHAPS is a long term programme which has
evolved throughout its period of implementation. Therefore
the question, 'What is CHAPS?' is important in establishing a
basis from which to begin evaluation work.

In initial CHAPS documentation four objectives were set for

the programme (Terrence Higgins Trust, unpublished tender document, 1996):

- to increase the focus on applied epidemiology, both geographically and by community, in developing and targeting health promotion messages;
- to enhance the links between applied research and HIV health promotion programmes for gay men and bisexual men, in the development and targeting of initiatives, as well as the evaluation of their effects;
- to expand the coverage of HIV health promotion work, targeting those poorly served by HIV health promotion work including men from black and Asian communities, bisexual men, and men with HIV;
- to enhance the cost effectiveness of health promotion for gay men and bisexual men in England.

Overall, it was expected to conform to the Health Promotion Strategy of the Terrence Higgins Trust which held as an objective 'to halve HIV acquisition by gay men and bisexual men' (Terrence Higgins Trust, 1995). Early on in the partnership, the latter objective was felt not to be feasible for the partnership, and, through discussion, CHAPS partners developed an alternative objective, 'to reduce the incidence of primary HIV infection in England resulting from sex between males'. Discussion about this led to the formation of a separate sub-group within the partnership, the Strategy Development Group, which produced the document *Making it count* (Terrence Higgins Trust, 1998). This document helped to clarify what aims CHAPS had. However, certain questions were left unresolved, including the extent to which *Making it count* is to inform working arrangements, including contractual arrangements and evaluation of the first phase of CHAPS and to what extent CHAPS should aim for wider implementation. These are fundamental questions in terms of what CHAPS is intending to do and which agencies CHAPS is seeking to influence.

What CHAPS is, what objectives it has, and what is important about it, have been shifting throughout the duration of the contract. This was probably a function of a number of factors, both positive and negative. There was a perceived lack of clarity at the outset about what the detailed aims and objectives of CHAPS were. On a more positive level, it represented the fact that CHAPS as a programme had developed in line with the concerns of partners such that descriptions of CHAPS from early literature were not representative of what partners wanted CHAPS to be by September 1997.

'It could have stayed just this number of outputs and different partners doing different pieces of work and a certain amount of communication. Like the shell, you look at the shell of the contract with the Department of Health, it's totally different to what the actual meat is now . . .' (CHAPS Project worker, March 1998)

This shift in the purpose of CHAPS made the work of evaluating it difficult. It is not easy to measure whether or not CHAPS has worked because it is not clear what it was trying to do. Partner agencies, in the interviews given for the process evaluation, referred to a different set of criteria for assessing CHAPS, based on their own opinions about the smoothness of the work, and their working relations. These substitute objectives may be wholly valid for workers or the agencies for which they work. They may also have validity in terms of health promotion or health gain. However, their importance is probably better acknowledged within the context of a systematic framework of aims and objectives.

The illuminative process evaluation enabled us to track these shifting objectives and to extrapolate the development of programme objectives from the other criteria for the success of the programme which were being used by project workers. In doing this, it enabled a more complete evaluation, under the conditions of constant change, than would have been possible by a fixed evaluation approach, using only initial project documentation.

Changing structures in the CHAPS partnership

The final challenge facing the evaluation work was the shifting structure of the CHAPS programme (Stewart *et al.*, unpublished report, 1998). Changes were manifest across the whole programme of work, and also in terms of the structures and organizations that impacted on the CHAPS programme. For example, a number of consultation groups representing all those partners who wished to take part were set up to provide direction to aspects of national programme work including mass media campaigns. A steering group was formed to provide guidance to the project, in place of the partnership weekends. New partners were added to CHAPS, and the role of some partners was changed from that originally envisaged.

Perhaps more significantly, the remit of the work of CHAPS also changed with the development of the strategy document *Making it count*, which meant that the way in which agencies outside the partnership used CHAPS resources became part of the objectives of the programme.

The process evaluation work was faced with a need to map these structural changes in the programme, and also to consider methods by which the broader scope of CHAPS work could be assessed.

A model for process evaluation in project implementation

Process evaluation has a valuable role to play during project implementation. It can help to clarify the structures and objectives of a health promotion programme, to provide a basis for outcome and final programme evaluation. It can also reflect back to project workers so that they get a history of the work they have been doing, to track shifts in project principles. It can usher in a culture of reflexivity whereby project workers have an opportunity to consider the broader health promotion approaches being used in the work they are doing, and it can give them a way of challenging these approaches. It can also help to reduce conflict within a programme.

In order to do any of these things, thought should be given to the way in which the process evaluation is organized and reported back to those who take part. If this is not done, then a process evaluation can cause conflict and weaken the programme it is intending to serve. The following points are necessary elements for the implementation of process evaluation.

Relationship with personnel

The evaluation should be able to gain trust among all the personnel involved in the programme and to report on their perspectives equally. This means that all partners should be involved in the evaluation, and regard it as a forum in which their opinions will be valued. Data should be meaningful to all the partners concerned, and useful for their health promotion work. It is important to explain the purpose of the evaluation and to negotiate feedback on the methods for data collection and reporting that are intended to be used.

Flexibility in programme design

Flexibility should be included in programme design, so that the results of the evaluation can be used to make meaningful changes to the programme. If such changes can only be made at certain times, under planning constraints, then these time constraints need to be made clear to project workers and evaluators.

Commitment of management

Related to the above point is the importance of a commitment from the agencies responsible for managing the project to use the results of the evaluation in making decisions. This will be dependent on them finding the evaluation useful and will therefore involve similar negotiations to those needed to gain trust on the part of project workers.

Mechanism for reporting back

There should be mechanisms to feed the findings of evaluation work back into decision-making systems within the project.

This involves plotting the time at which important project decisions are to be made, so that the evaluation can give an input into those decisions. Many projects will have constant rounds of decision making, and therefore it is important to decide in advance the points at which it is considered important for evaluation results to appear. This timeline should be agreed with all the workers taking part in the evaluation.

Methodological underpinning

For projects which are ongoing and have flexibility built in it is important that the evaluation uses methods which are able to provide reflexivity, so that it is able to track the development of a health promotion project from its beginning through changes that are made to the objectives or programme of work. This involves measuring the complex changes in the theoretical and methodological underpinnings of the project. A methodology is needed which can reflect this, and which can separate the day to day frustrations of project implementation from fundamental issues in health promotion.

Key points

- Process evaluation can assess whether the mechanisms of implementation were effective.
- In doing so, process evaluation can help explain why certain outcomes were achieved.
- Process evaluation draws on a number of research methods, both qualitative and quantitative.
- Process evaluation needs to be built in from the initial design of a project or campaign.
- Process evaluation needs to be carried out in partnership with all parties involved.
- Process evaluation needs to build in trust, reflexivity, and flexibility.

References

Aggleton, P. and Moody, D. (1992). Monitoring and evaluating HIV/ AIDS health education and health promotion. In *Does it work? Perspectives on the evaluation of HIV/AIDS health promotion* (ed. P. Aggleton, *et al.*) p. 16. Health Education Authority, London.

Hickson, F., Davies, P., and Weatherburn, P. (1997). Community HIV/AIDS prevention strategy: research and development review 1997. Unpublished. CHAPS, London.

King, E., Rooney, M., and Scott, P. (1992). HIV prevention for gay men: a survey of initiatives in the UK. North West Thames Regional Health Authority HIV Project, London.

Prout, A. and Deverell, K. (1995). Working with diversity: evaluating the MESMAC project. Health Education Authority, London.

Stewart, W., Wellings, K., and Malcolm, A. (1998). Community HIV and AIDS prevention strategy: third process report and interim evaluation report. Unpublished report. London School of Hygiene and Tropical Medicine Sexual Health Programme.

Terrence Higgins Trust (1995). *Health promotion strategy 1996–2001.* Produced by the Health Promotion Section of the Terrence Higgins Trust, Gray's Inn Road, London.

Terrence Higgins Trust (1996). Unpublished tender document for the research and development component of the CHAPS programme. Gray's Inn Road, London.

Terrence Higgins Trust (1998). Making it count: An Ethics, Theory and Evidence Based Health Promotion Strategy to Reduce the Incidence of HIV Infection through Sex between Men in England. Produced by the Strategy Development Group of the Community HIV and AIDS Prevention Strategy, Terrence Higgins Trust, Gray's Inn Road, London.

Windsor, R., Baranowski, T., Clark, N., and Cutter, G. (1994). *Evaluation of health education and disease prevention programmes.* Mayfield, Mountain View, California,.

8

Evaluating the use of public health risk factor simulation models

Bhash Naidoo

Usually the effectiveness of different intervention strategies is evaluated by experimental or observational methods in longitudinal studies such as randomized control trials, or cohort studies, the results of which would be extrapolated to estimate the effect for a given population. Unfortunately the time scales necessary for such studies can be prohibitive. This is particularly true for health promotion strategies which target risk factors for diseases with long latency periods, such as coronary heart disease (CHD). Current health care demands require policy decisions to be based on evidence, but the decisions must be made before there is time to collect evidence from observational studies.

In recent years the use of simulation models has been seen as a partial solution to the problem of the evaluation of health interventions, particularly in terms of interventions aimed at reducing the risk of non-communicable diseases (Manton and Stallard 1988; Morgenstern *et al.* 1992). These computer models allow policy makers to simulate the effects of different scenarios within a population, using available data on existing risk factor prevalence, the related relative risks of disease mortality, and the likely change in risk factor prevalence due to interventions, and then to project the results over several generations. It is envisaged that these models will be useful in evaluating the relative health gain of different approaches to attaining specific health outcomes. These models also permit policy makers to apply epidemiology to decision making at a population level.

This chapter will describe and assess the use of public health models as a tool for evaluation. Two different designs of models for the simulation of CHD outcomes are compared and contrasted, and the overall utility of simulation models as a tool for evaluation is considered.

Risk factor simulation models

Risk factor simulation models use results from longitudinal studies to derive the probabilities of certain risk factors causing death from particular diseases, and then apply these to appropriate populations. Routine data are used to provide the base line population information. Such data include health surveys providing data on the percentage of the population exposed to risk factors, census data providing the sex and age structure of a population, as well as birth projections for the population, actuarial data yielding information on life expectancy, and mortality records providing data on the death rates. Once the prevalences of risk factors for certain diseases are known, as well as the number of deaths these risk factor distributions result in, it is possible to use computer models to estimate the effect of altering these risk factor distributions in terms of the change in the number of deaths that would result.

Relative risks, population attributable risks, and multiple logistic equations are used as the basis of many of these types of model (Chambless *et al.* 1990; Chang *et al.* 1990). They have previously been used to relate data from sub-population studies to an individual's risk of a particular health outcome, as with the Framingham equation for CHD (Anderson *et al.* 1990), the Dundee Risk Score for CHD (Tunstall-Pedoe 1991) and the British Regional Heart Study Risk Score (Shaper *et al.* 1987). However, these equations are not adequate on their own to predict how the demographic characteristics and risk factor profile of a population will determine the outcome of interventions on that population, since the age and sex distribution will dictate the number of people at risk of disease, and thus will influence the magnitude of the effect of interventions. Morgenstern *et al.* (1992) have proposed the following characteristics as essential for models that simulate health policy options:

- a time period during which risk factors may develop, latent periods before risk factors affect morbidity and mortality, and lag times during which risk factor changes translate into mortality reduction;
- multi-factorial risk factor/disease relationships, where one risk factor can influence several diseases, and one disease may be influenced by several risk factors;
- a demographic basis by which population changes within the simulation period can be considered.

In terms of CHD health policy few models conform to these criteria. This is partly because CHD, unlike cancer, is a complex multistage disease for which there are few registries, particularly in terms of morbidity measures such as incidence, recurrence, and survival (Marmot and Elliot 1992). Models which attempt to simulate risk factor interventions on CHD must rely on informed estimates of these measures due to the lack of data. As a result such models are difficult to validate externally (Morgenstern *et al.* 1992), and this raises questions concerning the appropriateness of using unvalidated models.

Validation

There is resistance to, and scepticism of, modelling in the realm of health policy. The main reason for this is the difficulty in being able to validate these models. The usual way of validating such a model would be by historical testing, for instance where the known changes in risk factor prevalences in the past would be simulated to check if the model produced current mortality patterns. However, this is not possible with a model such as the cell-based model, PREVENT, since the model cannot take into account the effect of the reduction in risk factors not included in the model, or improvements in medical treatment which increase survival. Instead the concept of 'face-validity' is used, where one must try to validate the parameters which are used in the model. Even this can be problematic, and one may have to use data from a different population, or only a sub-group of a population, which might be quite unlike the population to be modelled.

This highlights how important data are to these models. The models are only as reliable as the data that are input. In order to produce better models there is a need to collect data which are the most appropriate for the population to be modelled, especially in terms of morbidity measures such as disease incidence and prevalence which may not be available for the specific population to be simulated. A particular problem in simulating health promotion interventions is the accuracy of data on the effectiveness of interventions, in terms of what changes in risk factor prevalence are achievable and how long individuals will continue with these changes in behaviour. These data may be difficult to find, and assumptions may have to be made.

Due to the number of assumptions and the difficulty in validating such models, they should be used with care. It is not advisable to use them to simulate the absolute effect of single interventions viewed in isolation, but rather they should be used to compare the magnitude of the health gain resulting from different interventions, given the same underlying assumptions.

Cell-based models

Two types of CHD policy models are discussed. One is a cell-based model and the other is a micro-simulation model. Within a cell-based model the population is subdivided into cells, such as by age, sex, and risk factor exposure categories, and it is to these separate cells that specific probabilities of events are applied. Over a simulated period the events for all the cells are summed to produce outcomes for the whole population, such as disease-specific mortality rates for each age group in the population.

These models use less computer memory and processing time than the micro-simulation models described below, and can therefore be run on less powerful computers. For example, the Prevent cell-based model originally ran on an IBM PC with 640KB of RAM and a maths coprocessor running under MS DOS 2.0. In general cell-based models tend to be easier for a lay audience to use and understand than micro-simulation models.

However, the methodology of cell-based models inherently imposes restraints on the complexity of the model, since increasing the number of data sets, risk factors, diseases, disease/risk factor relationships, age groups, and exposure categories will produce unmanageably large matrices of cells, and this can be a major disadvantage. For instance, with Prevent, a risk factor with two exposure categories covering five age groups for both sexes and linked to one disease will produce 20 cells for the prevalence of the risk factor, and these are associated with 20 probabilities of disease mortality, which equals 40 cells in all. Doubling the number of age groups, exposure categories, and disease associations will produce 80 cells for the prevalence, each with two probabilities of disease mortality, which equals 240 cells in all.

Prevent: a cell-based model

Prevent is probably the most accessible of the simulation models, due to its menu driven interface (Gunning-Schepers 1989). The model was developed in the Netherlands in 1988. Prevent can evaluate the health benefits for a population of changes in risk factor prevalence due to both trends and interventions. This can be done both in terms of proportional changes in disease-specific incidence and in terms of absolute changes in such parameters as disease-specific and total mortality. The underlying methodology requires:

- the possibility that one risk factor affects several diseases, and that one disease is affected by several risk factors;
- a time dimension to simulate the reduction in excess risk after cessation of exposure to the risk factor;
- the interaction between the effect of the intervention and the demographic evolution in the population.

After the user has specified the risk factor to be intervened upon, the model first calculates the expected development of the risk factors due to reasons other than the intervention, using data on expected trends. These are referred to as the autonomous developments. Next the user specifies change in risk factor prevalences which will occur after the intervention, using data on the expected effectiveness of the interventions, and then the model calculates the development of risk factor prevalences due to the intervention and the trends. Next the model calculates the autonomous development of all other risk factors that share diseases with the intervention risk factors; for instance cigarette smoking is a risk factor for CHD, cerebrovascular accident, chronic obstructive lung disease, and lung cancer. Finally the results of the calculations are applied to two populations, one with only the autonomous developments, and the other with both the autonomous developments and the intervention effects. The differences between the two populations are attributed to the intervention, with the output given in terms of total and disease specific mortality.

The main drawback to Prevent is that it only gives results of modelling in terms of mortality. No output information is available on morbidity, or the costs of treatment.

Micro-simulation models

By contrast, micro-simulation models depend upon a Monte Carlo simulation, where each individual in a cohort is generated separately using a random process, and over the simulation period these individuals can be subjected to certain events, the probabilities of these events being drawn randomly from distributions. These models, unlike cell-based models, therefore have the capacity to absorb all the required risk factors and interdependencies. The models require powerful computers with large capacity memories, since the life of each individual in the population must be generated and stored. Statistics Canada run the micro-simulation model POHEM on a dual Pentium II 266 MHz with 132 MB DRAM, and a simulation of 100 000 individuals would take about half an hour. However, these technical constraints are becoming less of a problem as the capacity of readily available computers increases.

The Population Health Model (POHEM): a micro-simulation model

POHEM has been developed at Statistics Canada. It uses the micro-simulation technique to model the dynamics of multiple risk factors and major diseases, one of which is CHD, under various demographic and health-related processes for a heterogeneous population (Wolfson 1994). The model uses a Monte Carlo process to generate random life tables, where, within each year, an individual is randomly simulated to either die, become ill, or stay well. The probabilities of changing states are randomly drawn from age specific uniform distributions. This process is repeated a considerable number of times to produce a large synthetic cohort.

Within the disease process is the CHD module, which uses Weinstein's Coronary Heart Disease Policy Model (Weinstein *et al.* 1987), originally a cell-based model, transformed to be consistent with the POHEM architecture, as well as using Canadian risk factor distributions and treatment protocols. The CHD module allows the user to simulate the effects of intervention, both preventive, by risk factor modification, and therapeutic, by changing case fatality rates, on mortality, morbidity, and costs over time. The CHD module is made up of three consecutive sub-models:

- The Demographic–Epidemiologic Model (DE Model), which generates disease free individuals, who are then aged. It uses a logistic risk function based on the Framingham equation to calculate the annual incidence rates of CHD events for each individual.

- The Bridge Model simulates the initial 30 days after the incidence of the first CHD event, with individuals having been passed on from the DE Model. First it determines the type of CHD event by age range and sex, then applies probabilities of death during the first 30 days following the event by age, sex, and type of event. A survivor then moves into the next sub-model.

- The Disease History Model classifies the individual with a previous CHD event into 12 CHD states. In each simulation year the patient is subjected to eight CHD event probabilities, which they may or may not experience, and each event and state have associated case fatality rates for CHD and non-CHD death, depending on disease history, age, and sex. These case fatality rates are applied to the individual to calculate those who survive to the next year of simulation and those who die.

POHEM does not need a large amount of computer memory to begin with since it avoids having to stratify the population by age, sex, and risk factor levels, in the way that is required in cell-based models. However, POHEM takes longer for a simulation run and requires substantial data storage space, due to its having to generate each individual of the cohort separately.

Overall the methodology of POHEM seems to give it great flexibility, since it has the ability to include external factors such as social status and environmental exposure, as well as the traditional risk factors. In addition the model seems to produce more detailed information on morbidity, in terms of functional and health status, and cost, in terms of health care utilization.

Targeting

These models allow the user to simulate the effect of targeting sections of a population, and so determine whether directing an intervention at one section of the population would produce more health gain than if it was directed at another, or to compare the effect of a high risk strategy to that of a population strategy (Rose 1992). For instance with a physical activity intervention it is possible to simulate the effect of targeting different age groups, or targeting individuals with a certain physical activity level (Naidoo *et al.* 1997). In addition modelling allows one to simulate the effect of the same intervention in different populations, be it at an international or national level, and so be able to investigate how the demographic characteristics of a population can influence the effect of intervention.

Differences between the models

Although both models can be used to simulate the effect of risk factor interventions, they have inherent differences which affect the type of interventions they can simulate and how they simulate those interventions. These main differences are:

1. Prevent simulates the whole population while POHEM only simulates a birth cohort, and so it is not possible to simulate the effect of an intervention targeted at the whole, or part of, the population other than one birth cohort with POHEM.
2. Prevent uses independent risk factor distributions while POHEM uses the multi-variate distribution, which means that Prevent cannot simulate high risk intervention strategies that target those individuals who have a clustering of risk factors.
3. Prevent uses relative risks of CHD death while POHEM uses a logistic regression equation to calculate the probability of a CHD event, which means that POHEM can produce results in terms of morbidity and mortality measures whereas Prevent can only produce mortality measures.
4. Prevent can only simulate the effects of cessation of exposure to a risk factor while POHEM can simulate the effects of reducing exposure. This means that with Prevent it is impossible to shift the risk factor distribution, as would be the effect of a population intervention.

It is not possible or sensible to put these models into a hierarchy in which one model is better than the other. Prevent is better suited for simulating certain interventions, while POHEM is best suited for simulating others. The type of intervention that is to be simulated will dictate the type of model one will use.

So can models be used to evaluate health promotion interventions?

Currently policy decisions are being made with only limited experimental knowledge on the effect of interventions, and without any information on how these interventions affect specific populations. Models have the ability to use available data on the effectiveness of interventions linked to demographic data, and to project the effects over several generations. However, models are only a partial solution to the evaluation of health interventions, since they are still based on limited data and may not be possible to validate. Consequently, when using such models one must be aware of the limitations of the input data, and the assumptions underlying the methodology of the model and used in translating the intervention to the simulation environment. Most of all, one must be wary of over-interpreting the output. Models can be a useful tool for evaluation, as long as policy makers are fully aware that they simulate a simplified version of reality, and should be used with caution.

Key points

- Simulation models can be useful tools for the evaluation of interventions.

- The assumptions made in the simulation need to be considered when interpreting these models' outputs.

- The quality of a model is dependent on the quality of the data it uses.

- The intervention to be simulated will dictate the choice of model used.

- Simulation models are useful in comparing the magnitude of health gain resulting from different interventions rather than for calculating the absolute effect of single interventions.

References

Anderson, K. M., Odell, P.M., Wilson, P. W. F., and Kannel, W. B. (1990). Cardiovascular disease risk profiles. *American Heart Journal*, **121**, 293–8.

Chambless, L. E., Dobson, A. J., Patterson, C. C., and Raines, B. (1990). On the use of a logistic risk score in predicting risk of coronary heart disease. *Statistics In Medicine*, **9**, 385–96.

Chang, H.-G. H., Lininger, L. L., Doyle, J. T., MacCubbin, P.A., and Rothenberg, R. B. (1990). Application of the Cox Model as a predictor of relative risk of coronary heart disease in the Albany Study. *Statistics In Medicine*, **9**, 287–92.

Gunning-Schepers, L. J. (1989). The health benefits of prevention, a simulation approach. *Health Policy*, **12**, 1–256.

Manton, K. G. and Stallard, E. (1988). *Chronic disease modelling*. Griffen, London.

Marmot, M. and Elliot, P. (ed.) (1992). *Coronary heart disease epidemiology—from aetiology to public health*. Oxford University Press.

Morgenstern, W., Chigan, E., Prokhorskas, R., Rusnak, M., and Schettler, G. (ed.) (1992). *Models of noncommunicable diseases— health status and health service requirements*. Springer-Verlag, Berlin.

Naidoo, B., Thorogood, M., McPherson, K., and Gunning-Schepers, L. J. (1997). Modelling the effects of increased physical activity on coronary heart disease in England and Wales. *Journal of Epidemiology and Community Health*, **51**, 144–50.

Rose, G. (1992). *The Strategy of preventive medicine*. Oxford University Press.

Shaper, A. G., Pocock, S. J., Phillips, A. N., and Walker, M. (1987). A scoring system to identify men at high risk of heart attack. *Health Trends*, **19**, 37–9.

Tunstall-Pedoe, H. (1991). The Dundee coronary risk-disk for management of change in risk factors. *British Medical Journal*, **303**, 744–7.

Weinstein, M. C., Coxson, P. G., Williams, L. W., Pass, T. M., Stason, W. B., and Goldman, L. (1987). Forecasting coronary heart disease incidence, mortality, and cost: the coronary heart disease policy model. *American Journal of Public Health*, **77**, 1417–26.

Wolfson, M. C. (1994). POHEM—a framework for understanding and modelling the health of human populations. *World Health Statistics Quarterly*, **47**(3–4), 157–76.

Part III

Evaluation in practice

9

Evaluating mass media approaches

Kaye Wellings and Wendy Macdowall

Broad spectrum interventions, intended to reach the general population, make use of mass communicational approaches such as TV, radio, press, billboard posters, and leaflets. These media are important sources of health information. Not everyone can be reached through community approaches and high profile communication can reach hidden groups within the general population. Box 9.1 highlights some of the roles that the mass media can fulfil.

Box 9.1   The role of mass media

Mass communicational approaches can:

- reach a wide audience;
- reach hidden groups within the population;
- place the health issue on the public agenda;
- legitimate interventions at other levels;
- trigger other initiatives.

Evaluation is particularly important in the case of mass media interventions because of the high costs involved. Yet the problems inherent in evaluation of all health promotional activities are exacerbated in broad spectrum approaches. The major strength of the mass media (their ability to reach a wide audience) paradoxically presents the greatest challenge for evaluation. Whereas the target audience of an intervention using a formal educational or clinical setting is more easily followed up, surveillance of the mass audience is difficult. There is less control over the destination and reception of preventive messages and thus they may fail to reach audiences for which they were intended, or they may reach audiences for which they were not intended and may be misconstrued. Furthermore, mass media interventions may have unintended consequences over which health promotion agencies have little control.

Two important themes are of particular concern in the context of mass media interventions:

- *Observed effects will be smaller.* Broad spectrum interventions do not target high risk individuals who have greater scope for change. Change at the level of a large and undifferentiated population is likely to be smaller.
- *Effects are more difficult to attribute to mass media intervention.* Attributing outcomes to a specific intervention is complicated where mass communication techniques are used. An effective campaign will have an effect far beyond its original remit, creating media discussion, providing the impetus for local efforts, and so on. The effects of the intervention are not easily distinguished from other events concurrent with it, or subsequent events triggered by it.

The scope of interventions: individual change and social diffusion

The strength of mass media, according to some, lies in helping to place issues on the public agenda and in legitimating local efforts, raising consciousness about health issues, and conveying simple information (RUHBC 1989; Tones *et al.* 1990). What the mass media do less effectively is to convey complex information, teach skills, shift attitudes and beliefs, and change behaviour in the absence of other enabling factors.

Two models are applicable in the evaluation of mass media interventions. The first, the 'risk factor' or epidemiological model is principally concerned with changing individual health-related behaviour, based on the premise that this will change health status. The second, the 'social diffusion' model, has more to do with the process of intervention and its catalytic effect, and the interaction between the component parts (Rogers 1983). If mass media interventions are effective, it is likely to be because they activate a complex process of change in social norms rather than because they directly change the behaviour of individuals.

An explicit objective of many mass media campaigns, then, is to change the social context and to effect a favourable climate in which interventions could be received. The college principal/publican/garage proprietor, previously doubtful about the propriety of installing a condom machine in his sixth form college/pub/garage, feels reassured and validated by a government backed mass media campaign promoting condom use. The young person, motivated to use condoms by the same campaign, is further encouraged to do so by their ready accessibility in the college/pub/garage in which he studies/drinks/buys petrol. This is sometimes known as 'diffusion acceleration'

The discrete contribution of different components is difficult to assess. Influences on our behaviour are multiple and are as likely to counteract, as to be in unison with, health advice. The biggest changes in behaviour, and hence health status, are likely to come about through forces other than health promotional interventions. For example, smoking behaviour is determined by the price of cigarettes, restrictions on smoking in public places, and voluntary impositions of bans (for example by a member of household).

Because of the high cost of use of the mass media, a campaign of short duration can consume a large proportion of the funds available for preventive interventions. A valid aim therefore may be to prompt coverage of the campaign by the free media.

The evaluation process: stages of research

Evaluation research begins with a *developmental component*, in which the potential for intervention in any health problem is described, along with (wherever possible) identification of factors that might facilitate or obstruct the delivery. This is followed by a *formative evaluation* in which the candidate intervention is pre-tested. During the course of the delivery of the programme a *process evaluation* is undertaken and finally, an *outcome evaluation* is carried out, which examines effects, effectiveness, and efficacy. If effectiveness is demonstrated and the service continues, routine monitoring and audit subsequently ensure quality of service delivery and continued efficacy.

A circular process

Development of the research and evaluation process is optimally seen, not as linear, but circular, that is, data from the outcome stage of evaluation will feed back into development of interventions, closing the 'loop'. Subsequent generations of programmes will benefit from insights into the effectiveness of the previous one. An important function of evaluation is to provide a means of detecting and solving problems and planning for the future. Providing retrospective feedback on success or failure at the end of an intervention provides guidance when it is too late to do anything about it. Ideally, the process should be continuous, tracking the progress of initiatives over time and feeding back information that can help operational decision making (see Chapter 7).

Formative research

Formative research involves exploratory work to guide the design of the intervention. An important component is the pre-testing of materials, as there is potential for messages to be misunderstood. It is important to know whether an intervention failed in its mission because it was not heard, or because it was not understood. Formative research, which typically uses focus groups (see Chapter 5), is useful in checking that an audience understands the language and images used.

Box 9.2

A series of AIDS public service announcements run by the UK Health Education Authority in 1988 aimed to convey the message that adoption of risk reduction practices needs to be universally applied because of the difficulty of distinguishing between those with and without the virus. The advertisement (Fig. 9.1 below) attempted to show that there were rarely visible symptoms of AIDS and that those with HIV have the same facial features as those without. No problems in relation to clarity of the message were revealed during pre-testing, but independent research by academic media analysts revealed considerable misinterpretation, with some believing the advertisement to be attempting to convey an accurate impression of what someone with HIV looked like (Kitzinger 1991).

The formative phase of evaluation aims to anticipate possible unforeseen outcomes. These are often favourable. For example, as a result of AIDS education using mass media interventions, the ruling on TV advertising of condoms was changed in several countries, including France, the UK and Ireland (Wellings and Field 1996). But they may also be unfavourable. A controversial press advertisement had the message that we should not take the numbers of people with AIDS as an indication of the scale of the problem, but rather the number of those with HIV. It posed the question 'What is the difference between HIV and AIDS?' and provided the answer 'Time'. Pre-testing showed the advertisement to convey the intended message effectively. The pre-testing research was conducted amongst the target audience of those who were uninfected, and could not predict the ensuing storm of protest from people with HIV. It proved an insensitive message with dire consequences for those affected, and was conse-

Fig. 9.1 How to recognize someone with HIV. (Copyright Health Education Authority.)

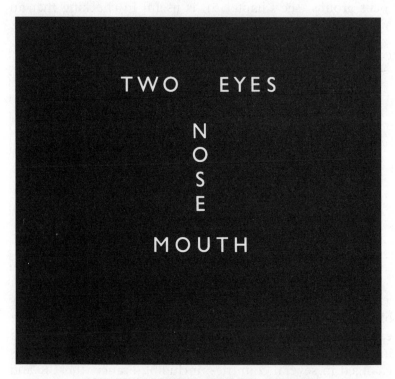

TWO   EYES

N
O
S
E

MOUTH

**HOW TO RECOGNISE SOMEONE WITH HIV
(THE VIRUS THAT LEADS TO AIDS).**

We all know how devastating the effects of AIDS can be.

But what are the signs of the Human Immunodeficiency Virus, the virus that leads to AIDS?

The fact is, a person can have HIV for years without the signs developing. During this time they may look and feel perfectly healthy.

But through sexual intercourse, they can pass on the virus to more and more people.

Already there are many thousands of people in this country who are unaware that they have the virus.

Obviously the more people you sleep with the more chance you have of becoming infected. But having

fewer partners is only part of the answer.

Safer sex also means using a condom, or alternatively, having sex that avoids penetration.

HIV is now a fact of life.

And while infection may be impossible to recognise, fortunately it is possible to avoid.

AIDS. YOU'RE AS SAFE AS YOU WANT TO BE.

quently withdrawn. Formative evaluation should take place with both target and non target groups.

Process evaluation

Research should be capable of revealing not only *whether* a campaign has succeeded but *why*, so that the findings can be used to guide future developments. Process evaluation is often narrowly conceived in terms of measuring 'dose' or exposure—either objectively in terms of the extent to which the campaign was aired (number of TV spots; broadcasting times; frequency and duration; audience figures; numbers of posters/ leaflets displayed) or subjectively (TV spots seen; time spent watching; time spent reflecting; level of interest) and in this sense more closely resembles audit.

While outcome evaluation focuses on the goals of a programme, process evaluation is important in providing insights into what factors may hinder or facilitate their achievement (see Chapter 7). Potentially favourable effects of a campaign can be seriously attenuated by an adverse response. By definition and design, exposure to the mass media is universal. Tailoring messages to specific target groups is less easily

---

Box 9.3

Specific issues to be addressed in *process evaluation* include:

- How well were resources allocated and disseminated?
- Were there any adverse side effects of the intervention?
- Was there harmony between the aims of health promotion and the needs of clients?
- Were there social and political dynamics that interfered with the ways in which health educational messages were received and responded to?
- Were there alliances between different interventions or environmental factors which enhanced outcomes?

achieved and problems of social and political acceptance can arise where messages are seen by those for whom they were not intended. Process evaluation also has valuable potential in helping to uncover unintended consequences of intervention.

Outcome evaluation: does it work?

Two key criteria for outcome evaluation are the size of effect and the possibility of attributing the outcome to the intervention. On both of these criteria, mass media work is problematic for evaluation.

Size of effect

The size of the expected effect is often not specified in the intervention plan, but a vital question is how large the effect has to be in order to make the case for the intervention having worked. Gains made in the case of mass media interventions may be modest because of:

- *The size of the target population*   Effects will be smaller where the target group is a large and heterogeneous mass.
- *The nature of outcome measures or endpoints*   Changes may be small because the wrong level of objectives has been chosen. Where measures of morbidity and mortality are used as outcomes in interventions aimed at the general population the sample needs to be impossibly large, and the scale of effect may still be too small to interpret.
- *The scope of the intervention*   Little effect may be seen because the endpoints are too narrowly conceived in terms of individual behaviour. Procedures need to be developed which attempt to measure effectiveness in terms of changes wrought in the social context.
- *The time scale*   The time scale looked at may be too short. Health promotional efforts must be of long duration to have significant effects. Despite being small scale, initial differences may be sustainable. The 30-year anti-smoking campaign in the United States is an excellent example of the potential of such sustained efforts.

Some of these issues are dealt with below, under the heading *Selection of indicators or outcome measures*. Although difficult to interpret, small effects may be of greater consequence where large numbers of people are involved and, even if unpromising when looked at from an individual perspective, can be important in public health terms. It is at the level of subgroup activity that achievements become observable, hence the importance of disaggregating data by groups of interest.

Attributing outcome to intervention

A major challenge in assessing efficacy of mass media approaches to prevention is that of attributing outcome to intervention, that is, ensuring that the observed effects are truly the outcome of public education campaigns and not the result of *a priori* differences or differential exposure to something else, such as the mass media generally or local preventive interventions.

The evidence is that hybrid interventions seem to work better than those with only one component, and the success seems to lie in the interaction effects between component parts. A valid goal for an intervention may be not to initiate trends in behaviour, but to accelerate those already existing. The effects may be enhanced by synergy; where there are multiple coinciding influences on behaviour, the outcome is likely to be more marked. 'Background noise' is often considered problematic in the context of outcome evaluation. The task of outcome evaluation is to look at the extent to which a mass media intervention is successful in harnessing environmental influences to its aims. Instead of trying to disentangle the variables, efforts need to be made to quantify the interaction effects. It may be beyond the power of an evaluation to determine which elements of the programme were effective. Moreover, it is likely to be misleading to attribute, to a particular focused action, an effect which may well have been the product of a complex mobilization producing norm change. Evaluation efforts need to find ways of measuring the catalytic effect of mass media interventions.

Selection of indicators or outcome measures

Outcome evaluation requires the use of indicators by which the outcomes can be measured. Conventionally, outcome measures are determined by the objectives of interventions. Lack of clarity regarding the objectives of the mass media intervention is a common problem for their evaluation. Setting objectives at an inappropriate level can threaten the apparent success of the intervention. In most cases, the proximate outcome variable in the biomedical model will be the adoption and maintenance of behaviours that reduce risk and these may constitute the indicators themselves (for example condom use, increased uptake of immunization, change in drinking/smoking habits). Intermediate outcomes (for example serum cholesterol levels, weight) relate more indirectly to the goals of intervention. The more distal variables—incidence of disease, morbidity, or mortality are not sensitive indicators for the general population, for reasons already discussed. Outcomes relating to proximate points along the causal pathway—awareness of risk, intention to change, modification of attitudes, are more feasible but less attractive in terms of 'proof' of effectiveness, while distal endpoints are more attractive in terms of scientific rigour, but success in achieving these goals will be remote.

In practice, a variety of outcome variables is needed, some proximate to the intervention, others more distal. However, the majority relate to intermediate objectives that will be achieved along the way; the assumption being that all these outcomes are related causally. For example, for a mass media campaign to increase uptake of immunization, valid proximate outcome measures would include attitudes towards, and knowledge of, the relevant health services; the intermediate indicator would be attendance uptake of immunization; and the distal outcome would be a reduction in incidence of infectious diseases. The link between the different outcomes in terms of health status must be made explicit.

The social diffusion model of health promotion has implications both for the size of the effect needed and for attributing outcome to intervention. Effects may be achieved which at the outset appear small, but there may be greater scope for them to be sustainable because the intervention has triggered a process of diffusion. A time element therefore needs to be built into the intervention.

Measuring unintended consequences

Operating within narrow bounds of a 'goal directed' model of evaluation will miss possibly adverse outcomes. Prior identification and definition of all the outcome variables may result in unforeseen and unintended effects going unrecognized and unrecorded.

Selection of research design

The question 'What are the methodological approaches which will allow us to support or reject claims of success?' follows logically from the question of how success can be measured. The options in terms of experimental approaches which can be applied to the evaluation of mass media interventions include lagged exposure or phased implementation (staggering interventions over time); area comparisons (comparing areas with and without interventions); and the application of media weight bias (comparing populations exposed to media interventions with those not so exposed).

Some would argue that the only legitimate goal of evaluation is to assess efficacy using experimental methods. Randomized controlled trials (RCTs) are probably the most rigorous methods of evaluation, but they will not be applicable in every case. The success of the experimental approach depends on being able to ensure that observed differences in outcomes between treatment and control group do not arise from any other factors than the intervention under investigation. Added to the problems of RCTs identified by Thorogood and Britton (Chapter 4) there are others which are either accentuated in the case of mass media interventions, or unique to them. Experimental approaches to evaluation are particularly poorly suited to interventions aimed at changing the social context. Some of the biggest influences on health related behaviours and health status occur at national levels. The broader the intervention, the more global its remit, the more far reaching its effects, the greater the interaction with other social forces and movements (and ironically the more interesting the outcome), the less amenable it is to a randomized controlled trial.

The problems of research design for mass media evaluation are:

- *Generalizability*   Campaign effects may be dependent on local circumstances that may not be generalizable to other areas or in the future.
- *Specificity*   Experimental and quasi-experimental designs are difficult to apply to mass media campaigns because ideally and by definition virtually everyone is exposed to them.
- *Comparison group*   Mass media interventions have problems identifying and maintaining the integrity of a comparison or control group. Many people and behaviours are not amenable to random allocation.
- *Size of effect*   The tendency to use relatively high discount rates (see Chapter 6) in the evaluation of health programmes does not favour health promotion programmes using the mass media. Large RCTs do not meet the first of the two criteria set out above (that is, that sufficiently large effects be observable). Little effect is likely to be seen, with the consequence that a given intervention is not replicated. Where there is a great deal of background communication going on, the intervention may provide only a very small increment.
- *Contamination*   The image of pristine treatment and control communities associated with the notion of the controlled trial is a false one. Trials attempting to give a communication treatment to one place and not to a neighbouring place ignore the social process at work.

Practical, ethical and, in some cases, economic obstacles may also impede the implementation of experimental strategies.

Alternative approaches

There is little point in finding out whether an intervention works better than another or none at all until we have first established what effects it has and whether it is effective, that is, whether it meets the objectives set for it. Any effects of an intervention need to be measured in order to assess whether there are, in addition to those intended, effects that are unintended and possibly adverse. Similarly, if the intervention fails to achieve the goals set for it, the question of whether it did so more cost-effectively than another or none at all will be irrelevant.

Programmes using the mass media should be evaluated with a methodology which respects their character and the way they work, but is credible enough to influence policy decisions. An eclectic approach to research and evaluation is called for. In the words of the late Geoffrey Rose, we need researchers with 'clean minds and dirty hands'. Alternative approaches, including natural experiments, correlated time series, and other non-experimental and quasi-experimental approaches are needed.

Measures of Effect

Several methods have been used to measure effects and effectiveness.

Retrospective reporting In this, respondents are simply asked if they have gained in knowledge, changed their attitudes or modified their behaviour. This method may be the only available in many cases, yet, because of the absence of baseline data, suffers from biases introduced by desirability response and recall difficulties.

Longitudinal designs These have advantages over a cross-sectional design and are more appropriate to understanding the process of behaviour change. Panel studies have disadvantages of attrition yet these may be balanced by the advantages of knowledge of behaviour prior to the intervention.

Time series data   Evaluation of effectiveness typically uses a pre- and post-test design and these methods are less complex and less costly than RCTs. Time series data use narrative to make the case for observed effects being attributable to the intervention—the equivalent of 'telling a story with data'. Ideally, interrupted time series data are needed, that is, before and after intervention. Pre- and post-test surveys and tracking surveys offer some improvement over one-shot studies but are still susceptible to desirability response and provide no assurance that what is being measured is the effect of a particular intervention and not a generalized response to the health issue.

Correlated time series   Correlated time series data, using pre- and post-test data and statistical modelling techniques, help trace the causal pathway to the objectives, identifying intervening variables, and they also control for a number of problems of inference. Strength of effect and absence of confounding are taken as credible evidence that what mattered in interpreting effects was the intervention rather than there being a need for an *a priori hypothesis*. Structural equations, used to examine the direct effect of the intervention, and also the indirect effect on intervening variables though the use of regression models, are able to assess the strength of each of the factors. They may be more appropriate than RCTs in the context of evaluation of mass media interventions because of their ability to assess the relative effect of more than one antecedent variable on outcome and, conversely, to assess how much of the effect was attributable to particular influential factors.

Knowledge, attitude, and behaviour (KAB) surveys

Survey investigation is the mainstay of data collection procedures. Typically, KAB surveys are used which investigate exposure to, recall, and comprehension of campaign messages and self reported behaviour change. KAB surveys have limitations in the extent to which they can monitor changes wrought in the social context, since their focus is on the individual. They also present problems of validity and reliability and are susceptible to social desirability response.

Triangulation

One solution to the problem of bias in the data collecting process has been to attempt to triangulate results, or to cross-validate against other data sources which might provide more objective measures of behavioural change. A good deal of information is available at relatively low cost and might include a selection from the following: sales figures (of, for example, cigarettes, alcohol, condoms, low fat spreads), subscriptions to exercise classes or health clubs, immunization uptake, screening uptake (for example mammography, HIV test data), helpline statistics, morbidity and mortality data, and media reports. The combination of behavioural and clinical measures offers potential for triangulation, helping to verify inferences drawn from self reported data, despite methodological and scientific difficulties.

Media analysis

As noted above, programmes may work because they activate a complex process of change in social norms rather than because they produce behaviour change directly at the level of the individual. Media analysis provides a valuable indicator of changes in the social context. This requires the use of a reputable media cuttings audit agency, or assiduously keeping a cuttings file. Where the intervention is under trial in one region, such that one area receiving the intervention is compared with another which does not, local media audit is particularly important.

Independence of the evaluation team

The choice of agency to carry out the evaluations is pivotal in determining the quality of the data produced, the manner in which it was used, and its impact on future campaigns. There is clearly a political dimension of evaluation since it may show projects as not as effective as the originators believed they would be. Inevitably, where those commissioning the evaluation are also responsible for the campaigns, it is more difficult to ensure objectivity and impartiality.

Key points

Evaluation of mass media health promotion interventions must take account of the fact that such interventions:

- have effects beyond their original remit;
- influence the social context;
- reach groups and individuals outside of the target groups;
- may have unintended effects;
- should use a range of evaluative methods.

References

Kitzinger, J. (1991). Judging by appearances: audience understandings of the look of someone with HIV. *Journal of Community and Applied Social Psychology,* 1(2), 155–63.

Research Unit in Health and Behavioural Change (1989). *Changing the public health.* Wiley, Chichester.

Rogers, E. (1983). *Diffusion of innovations.* The Free Press, New York.

Tones K., Tilford, S., and Robinson, Y. (1990). *Health education, effectiveness and efficiency.* Chapman and Hall, London.

Wellings, K. and Field, B. (1996). *Stopping AIDS. AIDS/HIV and the mass media in Europe.* Longman and the European Commission, New York.

10

Evaluating community development initiatives in health promotion

Rachel Jewkes

Community development initiatives have become a familiar part of the repertoire of health promotion interventions. They involve active engagement with a fairly defined group of people over an extended period of time to explore their health and social needs, mobilizing available resources to meet these, usually improving primary health care services, and promoting healthier practices. Whilst the component activities within a community development initiative draw on other health promotion approaches, the intervention as a whole differs from these approaches in an important respect. In addition to benefits which may accrue from the outcomes of the component activities, the process of participation in the initiative is perceived to be in itself health generating (Vuori 1984). The arguments for community participation are summarized in Jewkes and Murcott (1998). Important amongst these is the belief that participation is empowering for participants, as it develops skills and competencies which can be applied to areas of life which extend well beyond the activities of a community development initiative. Furthermore, the process of engaging people in cooperation for mutual benefit generates social capital. Measures of this have been shown to predict age adjusted mortality rates (Wilkinson 1996). Evaluation of community development initiatives must therefore focus as much on the nature and extent of community involvement in the project as on the outcomes of the component activities and improvement in health. This chapter concentrates on the evaluation of community involvement. The evaluation of component activities is covered by other chapters in this book.

Evaluations of community development initiatives pose considerable challenges. These stem, in part, from the fact that the objectives and activities of an initiative are usually iterative in nature, there is no pre-defined end point or criteria for 'success'. Compound methodological problems, common to other health promotion evaluations, include the need for a mixture of methods, long time frames for health outcomes, and difficulties detecting moderate benefits when communities are small. In addition there is inevitably fluidity in the participant group and fluctuation in the nature of participation. Decisions about who to work with, and which projects, are strongly influenced by local, and sometimes national, political factors. It is these problems which form the core of this chapter, for whilst the notions of community, participation, and power have become common currency in health promotion literature, they are amongst the most hotly debated and contested ideas within the social sciences. Their operationalization within community development initiatives poses considerable theoretical and practical difficulties which are important because of the emphasis on evaluating process in this type of health promotion intervention.

Meanings of community

The search for an empirically based understanding of the nature of community has been a major theme in twentieth century sociology (Jewkes and Murcott 1996). By the 1960s sociologists had come to accept that an agreed and substantiated definition of community could not be attained. Nonetheless the literature relating to community participation is replete with normatively prescribed definitions. For example, Suliman (1983, p. 407) defines community as 'a group of people with a sense of belonging, with a common perception of collective needs and priorities and able to assume a collective responsibility for collective decisions'; Adams (1989) states that it should be defined 'geographically or as a community of interest for example a street, estate, women's group, black group, pensioner's group'. Frequently those engaged in community participation have reflected that what might be thought of as a community in definitions like the latter, do not match up to the former (Cutts 1985). In practice, therefore, normative definitions are at best a guide and those working in the area are forced to engage continuously with adjudication of competing meanings.

Some insights into how this is done can be found in the work of Jewkes and Murcott (1996), who studied community development initiatives in four districts in southeast England. They found 28 different types of definition of community within interviews discussing the projects. The constraints of funding and project management required each initiative to have a formal definition, for example 'everyone who lives and works in Westminster' or 'everyone who lives on a housing estate'. This described the boundaries of the community development initiative and the broad aim of the project was framed in terms of promoting health within this 'community'. Its definition was based on local authority and/or geographic boundaries, which were of importance with respect to access to resources. This definition was not perceived to be very relevant to the daily activities of most of the people working with 'the community'. Instead they constructed 'communities' for these purposes from sub-segments of this community, usually around a defining characteristic which suggested a particular type of need; for example adolescents in youth clubs might be a community for a drug use intervention or Kurdish women refugees for activities around women's health services. The relationship between these 'communities' and the formally defined one was described in terms of 'communities within the community'

The processes of operationalizing 'community' mean that instead of there being one community to consider in an evaluation, there are many. Each activity within a community development initiative will be organized with, and intended to impact on, a different sub-set of the population. This must be taken into account in evaluation. For each activity the relevant group must be defined and characteristics of participation and outcomes evaluated with respect to this. This is not to say that the formal definition of 'community' is never appropriate. Some interventions will be applied to the whole population, and the extent and nature of community participation in the community development initiative must be evaluated with respect to this. What is important is that evaluators question who is the appropriate target group for each aspect of the evaluation, rather than assuming that the formal definition of community is appropriate.

Who participates?

In constructing these smaller 'communities', health promoters implicitly recognize that what may be called a community within a community development initiative is a heterogeneous group with multiple, interrelated axes of difference, including wealth, gender, age, religion, ethnicity and, by implication, power. Indeed, Navarro (1984) suggests that a community should be regarded as a set of power relations within which people are grouped. Health promoters working in such environments are continuously faced with choices as to who to work with, be this through accepting an approach from a 'community' or through the deliberate selection of people as a collaborating group. These choices inevitably have consequences in terms of the dynamics of power at a local level and ultimately the ability of the initiative to maximize its potential impact in the population.

Steering committee membership and other participant roles

One set of decisions relate to the construction of steering groups for the initiative and often some of the sub-activities of the initiative. Projects may be most easily facilitated if organized through the medium of dominant local stakeholders or 'leaders', who are often most able to mobilize resources and articulate concerns. Yet the poorest and most marginalized are rarely represented amongst them. On the one hand, working through local power structures invites manipulation of the project according to the agendas of the powerful. On the other, working outside (and inevitably, potentially against) these structures can both weaken the potential impact of the project at a wider level and invite continued marginalization. Ideally the initiative's steering group should be broadly representative of the community, including both the most powerful and marginalized, but in practice this is rarely the case. Jewkes and Murcott (1998) found that in determining the membership of such steering groups practical concerns, such as whether someone had a telephone, or was available for meetings during the day, assumed a transcendence over all other considerations, including the extent to which different sectors of the population were reflected on the committee and any question of having a mandate to 'represent'. They found the 'community' to be represented almost exclusively by voluntary sector organizations and the representatives drawn from the funded elite of the voluntary sector. Thus even the representatives of the less powerful came from the most privileged quarters of that group. Other studies have shown that participants are usually people of higher income, educational level, and occupational group than average (Bates 1983, p. 16).

It is hardly surprising, then, that concern about the representativeness of representatives is a recurring theme within the evaluation of community development initiatives. Indeed, given the dimensions of difference within the community it is more surprising that anyone could consider that a small group of people could represent something as diverse as a notion of 'the community' than it is that those who try to do so are regarded as inadequate. Community representatives on steering groups should be chosen and valued for what they have to offer the group rather than perceiving them as representatives of an idealized 'community'. In this way their power bases can be recognized and biases acknowledged, rather than wished away.

Whether on the steering committee, or in the project as a whole, its important to recognize that not everyone within communities will be able to participate, nor will everyone be motivated to become involved (Seeley *et al.* 1992). Even if people are interested they may not be able to give the time. Participation is time consuming and often those who health promoters want to work with are too busy securing the necessities of life (Agudelo 1983). Considerable efforts are needed to involve marginalized groups. Participating communities are 'made not born'. Unless a definite commitment to working with the less powerful is part of the process, those who are relatively inaccessible, unorganized, and fragmented can easily be left out. Sometimes legitimate decisions must be made to exclude certain groups or individuals. In circumstances of extreme polarization, community development initiatives which have failed to acknowledge the reality of local politics have been turned into an arena for playing out macro-political struggles and have failed (Thornton and Ramphele 1989).

Evaluation and monitoring of who participates is essential, both at a steering committee level and in individual activities within the initiative, as many projects fail to engage non-elite groups (Reidy and Kitching 1986). Unless power dynamics are acknowledged in initiatives, there is a danger that engagement, particularly with more powerful groups, will result in initiatives intended to benefit those with greatest needs being used to their detriment (Nichter 1984).

Nature of participation

Once participation is secured, involvement in the research process is usually not continuous, not evenly sustained, nor predictable. Participatory theorists argue that participation can be best described as occurring in different degrees of involvement, often likened to the rungs on a ladder. Arnstein (1969) described eight rungs in descending order: citizen control, delegated power, partnership, placation, consultation, informing, therapy, and manipulation. The top three were described as degrees of citizen power, the middle three as degrees of tokenism, and the bottom rungs as non-participation. Although the ladder metaphor suggests some potentially orderly progression through these stages which might be achievable in a community development initiative, in practice different participants are likely to participate to different degrees. One participant may participate differently in different activities of the initiative or in different stages of one activity.

Where participation is largely towards the lower rungs, it is often perceived as primarily attributable to the lack of willingness of those with greater power, often the statutory sector, to concede power. It is also true that commitment and interest from community members waxes and wanes over time for a variety of reasons. Participants can experience task exhaustion and the composition of participating groups will fluctuate over time (Minkler 1992). Many people may be reluctant to invest their time and energy in the project particularly if it offers little in terms of direct or immediate benefit. Others may enter the participatory process with preconceived ideas of desirable outcomes. When it becomes apparent that these are not project priorities, their enthusiasm wanes. Local people may find that some of the needs which they identify are embraced with more enthusiasm and interest than others. For example, people are often encouraged to identify needs for primary health care but not for curative services. Practitioners need to tread a careful path between generating sufficient interest for participation and not raising false hopes. Identifying honestly the limitations of what can be achieved at the outset is an important part of establishing trust. This takes considerable time.

Evaluation of participation in the project as a whole and its individual activities must therefore look not just at the number and characteristics of the community members who are engaged, but also at the degree of participation. It needs to be done in a sufficiently complex manner to accommodate changes over time in different dimensions of the project. This is important both in ensuring that the objective of participation is achieved and that the extent of participation in activities is taken into account in the evaluation of their outcomes.

Whose views prevail?

In Suliman's (1983, p. 407) definition of community, cited above, notions of togetherness were central, and indeed many other authors (for example Cohen 1985) identify sharing characteristics, experiences, or views as a defining feature of community. It is not surprising that people engaged with health promotion do so, too. This becomes a problem in community development because a critical distinction needs to be recognized between communities constructed by their members (that is, those people who we think we share things with) and those constructed by non-members (that is, people who are assumed to share things). During the course of implementing sets of health promotion activities the boundaries of the 'communities' who are the targets are invariably determined by non-members. The boundaries of sharing are therefore assumed.

Within any local area people associate through multiple, overlapping networks with diverse linkages based around different interests. Isolated axes of difference, such as age or gender, are insufficiently sensitive as determinates of shared experience for coherent priorities to be identifiable among groups defined in this way. Health promoters find that competing, contested, and changing versions of 'community needs' or 'values' emerge according to the way in which their intentions are interpreted by these groups. These generate not only different interpretations but reveal different agendas and means for enacting some solutions and blocking others.

Caution is needed even when apparently coherent expressions of community needs or priorities are articulated; 'we think ...', 'we want ...' may reflect a significant distortion of an individual's aspirations. The very act of the 'community' engaging with outsiders necessitates a simplification of their shared experiences into a form and generality which is intelligible to the outsider. This simplification may imply notions of sameness which border on fiction and would not pass within the community (Cohen 1985). In the process of evaluation, health promoters need to continuously reflect on whose view is prevailing or whose needs are being expressed, what may be motivating this, and what alternative sets of needs and priorities might have been chosen.

A further consequence of assumptions of sharing is the idea, usually implicit, that benefits of an intervention, particularly political skills derived from participation, will diffuse within the community and in some way impact upon a broader group of people than those who are directly involved. This assumption is almost never evaluated, but the extent to which this occurs should be considered in the evaluation. It is important for evaluation to determine the number of people reached through an initiative.

Conclusions

Community development initiatives are characterized by multi-faceted interventions, with participation and joint working sought in the project as a whole and in the constituent activities. Evaluation of these projects must also be multi-faceted and specifically tailored to each part of the broader initiative. Definition of the population of relevance for each intervention, and evaluation of its impact in that group, is essential. Evaluation and monitoring of participation is important, as the process of participation is perceived to be health generating. This evaluation needs to be undertaken with particular reference to three questions: Who participates? What is the nature of that participation? Whose views prevail?

Key points

- A consensus on what is 'community' cannot be achieved, it must be defined specifically for each project evaluation.

- Without targeted effort to reach disadvantaged groups, only the more advantaged participate in community development initiatives.

- Evaluation should acknowledge that consistently high levels of participation by all players are not achievable, but the nature of participation at different stages of the project should be examined.

- Evaluation should not require that representatives on steering groups are 'representative', but should consider why they were chosen and whether it was appropriate.

- Evaluation should consider how decisions are made within projects and whose views prevail in these processes.

References

Adams, L. (1989). Healthy cities, healthy participation. *Health Education Journal*, **48**, 178–82.

Agudelo, C. A. (1983). Community participation in health activities: some concepts and appraisal criteria. *Bulletin of the Pan American Health Organisation*, **17**, 375–85.

Arnstein, S. (1969). Eight rungs on a ladder of citizen participation. *AIP Journal*, **July**, 216–24.

Bates, E. (1983). *Health systems and public scrutiny*. Croom Helm, London.

Cohen, A. P. (1985). *The symbolic construction of community*. Routledge, London.

Cutts, F. (1985). Community participation in Afghan refugee camps in Pakistan. *Journal of Tropical Medicine and Hygiene*, **88**, 407–13.

Jewkes, R. K. and Murcott, A. (1996). Meanings of community. *Social Science and Medicine*, **43**, 555–63.

Jewkes, R. and Murcott, A. (1998). Community representatives: representing the 'community'? *Social Science and Medicine*, **46**, 843–58.

Minkler, M. (1992). Community organising among the elderly poor in the United States: a case study. *International Journal of Health Services*, **22**, 303–6.

Navarro, V. (1984). A critique of the ideological and political positions of the Willy Brandt Report and the WHO Alma Ata Declaration. *Social Science and Medicine*, **18**, 467–74.

Nichter, M. (1984). Project community diagnosis: participatory research as a first step toward community involvement in primary health care. *Social Science and Medicine*, **19**, 237–52.

Reidy, A. and Kitching, G. (1986). Primary health care: our sacred cow, their white elephant? *Public Administration and Development*, **6**, 425–33.

Seeley, J. A., Kengeya-Kayondo, J. F., and Mulder, D. W. (1992). Community-based HIV/AIDS research—whither community participation? Unsolved problems in a research programme in rural Uganda. *Social Science and Medicine*, **34**, 1089–95.

Suliman, A. (1983). Effective refugee health depends on community participation. *Carnets de L'enfance* **2**, **2**. In F. Cutts (1985). Community participation in Afghan refugee camps in Pakistan. *Journal of Tropical Medicine and Hygiene*, **88**, 407–13.

Thornton, R. J. and Ramphele, M. (1989). Community. Concept and practice in South Africa. *Critique of Anthropology*, **9**, 75–87.

Vuori, H. (1984). Overview—community participation in primary health care: a means or end? IV International Congress of the World Federation of Public Health Associations. *Public Health Review*, **12**, 331–9.

Wilkinson, R. G. (1996). *Unhealthy societies: the afflictions of inequality*. Routledge, London.

11

Evaluation of health promotion in clinical settings

Dominique Florin and Sarah Basham

In this chapter we first discuss some general issues pertaining to health promotion in clinical settings, then address some specific issues relating to evaluation. Evaluation case studies on the prevention of coronary heart disease (CHD) by health checks in primary care and on the prevention of depression are used to highlight some of the key points. The evaluation of health promotion is addressed from a different perspective than is taken in the rest of the book in that our starting position is that of a particular setting in which health promotion may take place. The different evaluative methods and health promotion approaches described elsewhere in the book apply, to a greater or lesser degree, to health promotion in clinical settings, but there are specific features which apply to health promotion in clinical settings and which make its evaluation unique—in particular the involvement of health professionals. Almost by definition this involvement implies a 'top down' approach and this may be considered antithetical to many of the principles of health promotion. Inevitably the involvement of health professionals has had a profound effect both on the definition of the aims and the assessment of outcomes of health promotion in clinical settings and on the types of interventions used. Health professionals conventionally see their role as concerned with *health care* rather than *health* and this may lead to a reductive approach to what are considered health promoting interventions. Moreover, health professionals traditionally define health as the absence of disease rather than in the more positive ways described in Chapter 1. This may lead to health professionals holding a narrower perception of health promotion than others involved in the discipline.

The principal type of health promoting activity likely to occur in clinical settings is interventions to prevent disease (sometimes classified into primary, secondary, and tertiary prevention). Such interventions may be traditionally medical, such as immunization, screening, or drug treatment, or they may involve individual educational interventions around promoting health, often related to lifestyle changes. Health professionals may also be involved in wider health promotion activities, such as community development or influencing health policies, although these are not, strictly speaking, health promotion in clinical settings. In addition to the obvious health care settings such as hospitals, clinics, and health centres, clinical health promotion may also occur in settings such as community pharmacies, schools, and occupational health settings. Considering this range of settings has implications for the approaches required for evaluation.

The rationale for health promotion in clinical settings

Over the past 30 years there has been an increase in proactive prevention and health promotion in clinical work. By definition, clinical settings attract individuals who are unwell and at such times individuals may be particularly receptive to health promotion interventions, especially those related to lifestyle changes. For instance a patient attending a doctor, nurse, or pharmacist for a chest infection may be more likely to respond positively to advice on smoking cessation. Paradoxically, clinical settings can also attract well populations which are in a sense 'captive' and thus ideal for preventive interventions such as screening, the success of which depends on high population coverage rates. Examples here might include pregnant women attending for antenatal care, children in a routine school health check, or simply patients attending their doctors for other reasons.

The system of primary care in the UK has been particularly attractive for health promotion. This is because the vast majority of the population is registered with a single general practitioner and the vast majority of these individuals attend their doctor's surgery in the course of three years (Stott and Davis 1989). This provides the opportunity for both systematic and opportunistic health promotion interventions. In the US, similar considerations apply with the growth of health maintenance organizations, some of which require annual screening check ups for membership and which restrict referral to specialist care, unless first referred by a family physician. Of course health promotion can also take place in secondary care settings, but inevitably applies to more selected populations. Training in health promotion has generally not been a prominent part of doctors' medical education. Thus they may not have appropriate skills to effectively intervene to change lifestyle behaviours. However, amongst the different categories of health care professional certain groups are considered as being particularly suitable for health promotion. In the UK, nurses and health visitors have been identified in this way. In part this reflects their training, but also their organization relative to other health care professionals such as doctors. In the UK, one of the reasons given for involving nurses rather than doctors in health promotion is that it is considerably cheaper to pay the former for these activities (Fullard *et al.* 1987).

Methodological implications of evaluation of health promotion in clinical settings

The above considerations have implications for the evaluation of health promotion in clinical settings. Because a range of different interventions are used, so must there be a range of different approaches to evaluation. Thus the evaluation of a childhood immunization programme would be very different from that of a programme to increase well-being in elderly cardiac patients. The former might rely on morbidity and mortality outcomes such as rates of disease in childhood and on process measures such as assessment of the cold chain and numbers of children vaccinated. The latter might use mortality and morbidity outcomes, but might also use quantitative and qualitative outcomes related to quality of life, as well as process measures assessing the impact of the programme. There are sound reasons why the evaluation of health promotion in clinical settings cannot rely solely on measurement of mortality and morbidity. These outcomes are often too long term or too infrequent to be viable end points. There may also be major problems in attributing causality, especially in non-randomized trials carried out against a background of secular trends. Furthermore, the desired outcomes are not necessarily limited to changes in mortality or morbidity. Other outcomes, such as changes in health related behaviours, are more difficult to measure reliably if they do not yield changes in morbidity or mortality in the short term. For instance, one approach to smoking cessation involves encouraging changes in views and beliefs before permanent smoking cessation actually occurs, and those attempting to stop smoking may succeed, then restart on several occasions before succeeding permanently (Prochaska and DiClemente 1983). All these stages of change should form part of an evaluation of smoking cessation, and more research is needed to develop reliable ways of measuring these attributes.

An important area of health promotion in clinical settings is screening. Increasing numbers of diseases and risk factors can be screened for. Among many examples are preconceptual and neonatal screening for genetic disorders, childhood developmental surveillance, screening for CHD or its constituent risk factors, and cervical and breast cancer screening. A number of well established programmes exist, but many have been criticized precisely because they were set up without adequate evaluation. Cochrane and Holland (1971) have suggested a list of seven criteria for the evaluation of any screening tests: simplicity of the test, acceptability to patients, accuracy, cost, precision, sensitivity, and specificity. What is important about this list is that it stresses not just the technical efficacy of screening tests but also other aspects such as patient acceptability, and costs relative to potential benefits or other health service interventions.

Organizational factors within clinical settings are as important to the success of interventions as other attributes such as efficacy. One particular problem relates to the fact that voluntary health promoting interventions have differentially attracted those at lower risk and therefore with lower need, leading to an 'inverse care law' operating. One example is the tendency for the UK cervical screening programme to miss out older women who are at greatest risk of cervical cancer. It has been shown that women who die of cervical cancer are much less likely to have **ever** been screened than the general population. Therefore it has been suggested that rather than concentrating on shortening the screening interval, it would be more beneficial at a population level to ensure that all women get screened at least once (Holland and Stewart 1990). A similar phenomenon was observed when voluntary health checks for CHD were introduced in UK general practice. Again patients most likely to attend were those at least risk of coronary heart disease: the so-called 'worried well' (Waller *et al.* 1990). Furthermore, it was shown that this inverse care law operated at an organizational and population level. Practices in areas with low mortality for CHD were more likely to offer these preventive services than those in areas of high mortality (Gillam 1992). The implication of these examples is that it is essential that evaluations of health promotion in clinical settings take into account the population characteristics of both those who are and are not reached by the intervention. Limiting evaluations to the characteristics of the intervention would miss this essential point.

Evaluations must address the costs and opportunity costs of health promotion interventions, that is, not just effectiveness but also cost-effectiveness (see Chapter 6). Any intervention in a clinical setting represents an opportunity foregone for another intervention and it is important to evaluate interventions in this light. Thus, increasingly, health economists have been involved in the evaluation of health promotion programmes. Organizational factors can significantly change the cost effectiveness of interventions. For instance, the cost effectiveness of interventions will vary depending on the relative costs of the clinical staff involved. As already mentioned, one of the reasons that nurses rather than doctors have been involved in clinical health promotion is that they are cheaper to employ. Cost effectiveness will also vary depending on the risk level of the populations involved. In some cases interventions directed at those at high risk may be more cost effective than clinical interventions directed at those at all levels of risk.

Many of the points mentioned above, and others, are demonstrated in the case studies on the evaluation of the 'health check' approach to CHD prevention and on the secondary prevention of depression (Boxes 11.1 to 11.3). In the 1980s and 1990s in the UK there was an increase in primary care based prevention, particularly directed at the primary prevention of CHD. CHD is a multifactorial disease but research on many unifactorial interventions such as smoking cessation advice or blood pressure control has shown these to be effective. The first case study looks at the evaluation of the 'health check' approach, that is, multifactorial interventions for the primary prevention of CHD. Depression is a common illness for which there are effective secondary prevention interventions. Two different evaluation approaches of two programmes to improve the recognition and treatment of depression are described in the second and third case studies.

These case studies illustrates some of the methodological complexities of evaluating prevention in primary care using an experimental design. It is important to include organizational and cost factors in the evaluation. There are limitations in using experimental designs for complex behavioural changes, and a qualitative approach may sometimes be preferable. Equally there is a need to include very broad concepts such as the role of clinical services in order to assess the value

**Box 11.1   Case study:
lessons from the evaluation of health checks
for prevention of coronary heart disease
in primary care in the UK**

In the mid 1980s, a project was set up to test a 'health check' model and demonstrated that a systematic approach by practice nurses could significantly increase recording of blood pressure, smoking, and weight in patient notes (Fullard *et al.* 1987). A limitation of this evaluation was that it could not demonstrate whether increased recording of risk factors was translated into improvements in CHD occurrence. Despite this, the approach was widely taken up in practices. In the late 1980s two further trials (called Oxcheck and FHS) were set up to test the outcomes of the health check model, that is, multifactorial primary prevention. Both were randomized controlled trials and the interventions were carried out by nurses specially trained on risk factors in middle aged patients in clinic rather than opportunistic settings (Family Heart Study Group 1994; Imperial Cancer Research Fund OXCHECK Study Group 1995).

Results from Oxcheck showed that the large numbers of new cases identified by the health check approach were likely to outstrip the resources available to manage them in most practices, whilst an important proportion of the practice population would not be reached. The FHS results showed that 27% of the at-risk population did not attend the intervention. These findings demonstrate the importance of evaluating the practical implications and the extent of coverage of interventions of any intervention.

The Oxcheck results suggested that the change in cholesterol could be projected to a 6% decrease in myocardial infarction in men and 13% in women. The FHS authors projected that their intervention could lead to a 12% decrease in coronary risk, on the crucial assumption of long term maintenance of risk factor changes. Although these projections seem important at a population level, the authors and other commentators interpreted the results as showing the *in*effectiveness of population screening, which would require considerable redistribution of resources to be implemented in general practices. There was disagreement both regarding the validity of the estimates of changes and their value (National Heart Forum 1995).

(*cont. on page 147*)

Box 11.1   Case study (*cont.*)

One approach to resolve this is economic evaluation. Further analyses have suggested that it is less cost-effective to provide blanket screening than to concentrate on groups at high risk, for example those with pre-existing disease, with elevated cholesterol levels, men rather than women, and older rather than younger populations (Wonderling *et al.* 1996). However, studies have not looked at the opportunity costs of concentrating on such activities at the expense of other general practice activities, which is an important factor in assessing the value of health promotion in primary care.

---

of health promoting activities within them. Despite being very well designed scientific studies, Oxcheck and FHS did not resolve the issue of the value of health checks for CHD prevention in primary care. Methodologically, these trials have a weakness in common with many other complex intervention

---

Box 11.2   Case study:
mental health promotion for depression in Sweden

In 1983–84 the Swedish Committee for Prevention and Treatment of Depression introduced an educational programme for all general practitioners on the Swedish Island of Gotland (Rutz *et al.* 1989). The primary goal was to increase knowledge about diagnosis and treatment of patients with affective disorders. The program was evaluated both as a 'before and after' design (see Chapter 4) and in comparison with the Swedish mainland. Routine data were collected on suicides, referrals to the local psychiatric department, emergency admissions, the quantity of sick leave, the quantity of inpatient care due to depression, and rates of prescription for psychopharmacological drugs. Data were compared for periods before, during, and after the intervention and in comparison with the Swedish mainland. One methodological problem with this approach is that an island population such as that found on Gotland may have different characteristics to communities on the mainland and these may have influenced findings of the study.

Box 11.3   Case study:
mental health promotion for depression in the USA

A different approach was used in the USA to evaluate the Depression: Awareness, Recognition and Treatment campaign. A controlled trial of the intervention was carried out by Callahan *et al.* (1994). The intervention aimed to educate primary health care physicians to improve their diagnosis and treatment of depression in the elderly. Each physician in the intervention group had a program of three educational visits. The outcomes measured were frequency of recording of depression, stopping medications that can cause or exacerbate depression, initiating antidepressant medication, and psychiatry referral. Changes in HAM-D and Sickness Impact Profile scores (standardized self reporting scales) were measured in the patients recruited. The results of the trial showed that physicians in the intervention arm were more likely to diagnose depression and prescribe antidepressants but there was no change in the stopping of causative medications or referrals to psychiatry. There was no significant difference between the two groups of patients in their self reported outcome ratings. This study highlights some of the problems when looking at outcomes. The intervention appeared to have improved diagnosis and treatment of depression, but there was no measurable improvement in the outcome for the patient.

---

trials, in that they do not allow examination of which aspects of their interventions did or did not work. This is a limitation of the 'black box' design of randomized controlled trials. Even for the same clinical problem, there is no single methodological approach. While a randomized controlled trial may seem more 'scientific', not all interventions in clinical settings are amenable to experimental evaluation. Different approaches each have their strengths and weaknesses.

Conclusions

The case studies presented here demonstrate many of the issues that apply to other health promotion interventions in clinical settings. A broad view of evaluation is necessary that will take into account many aspects of interventions, not just their technical efficacy. Outcomes must extend beyond quantitative measures of mortality and morbidity. Organizational issues are crucial. Evaluation designs may or may not be experimental. In general, health promotion in a clinical setting is more likely to be amenable to an experimental or even randomized controlled trial design than health promotion in other settings. Even so, to limit evaluations to such designs would be to miss out very significant aspects of interventions.

Key points

- Clinical settings are useful for health promotion interventions because they offer access to a large proportion of the population at times when people are more likely to be responsive to health promotion.

- A range of evaluation techniques can be employed in clinical settings, but such settings are particularly amenable to trials.

- The evaluation of health promotion in clinical settings would be improved if researchers specified detail of the activities in an intervention (opened the black box).

References

Callahan, C. M., Hendrie, H. C, Dittus, R. S., Brater, D. C., Hui, S. L., and Tierney, W. M. (1994). Improving treatment of late life depression in primary care: a randomised clinical trial. *Journal of the American Geriatric Society*, **42**, 839–46.

Cochrane, A. L. and Holland, W. W. (1971). Validation of Screening Procedure. *British Medical Bulletin*, **27**(1), 3–8.

Family Heart Study Group (1994). Randomised controlled trial evaluating cardiovascular screening and intervention in general practice: principal results of the British family heart study. *British Medical Journal*, **308**, 313–20.

Fullard, E., Fowler, G., and Gray, J. A. M. (1987). Promoting prevention in primary care. A controlled trial of a low technology, low cost approach. *British Medical Journal*, **294**, 1080–2.

Gillam, S. J. (1992). Provision of health promotion clinics in relation to population need: another example of the inverse care law? *British Journal of General Practice*, **42**, 54–6.

Holland, W. W. and Stewart, S. (1990). *Screening in health care.* Nuffield Provincial Hospitals Trust, London.

Imperial Cancer Research Fund OXCHECK Study Group (1995). Effectiveness of health checks conducted by nurses in primary care: final results of the OXCHECK study. *British Medical Journal,* **310**, 1099–104.

National Heart Forum (1995). *Preventing coronary heart disease in primary care. The way forward.* Report of an expert meeting. HMSO, London.

Prochaska, J. O. and DiClemente, C. D. (1983). Stages and processes of self change in smoking: towards an integrative model of change. *Journal of Consulting and Clinical Psychology,* **51**, 295–304.

Rutz, W., Walinder, J., Eberhard, G., Holmberg, G., von Knorring, A. L., von Knorrring, L., *et al.* (1989). An educational program on depressive disorders for general practitioners on Gotland: background and evaluation *Acta Psychiatrica Scandinavica,* **79**(1), 19–26.

Stott, N. C. H. and Davis, R. H. (1989). The exceptional potential in each primary care consultation. *Journal of the Royal College of General Practitioners,* **39**, 369–72.

Waller, D., Agass, M., Mant, D., Coulter, A., Fuller, A., and Jones, L. (1990). Health checks in general practice: another example of inverse care? *British Medical Journal,* **300**, 1115–18.

Wonderling, D., Langham, S., Buxton, M., Normand, C., and McDermott, C. (1996). What can be concluded from the Oxcheck and British family heart studies: commentary on cost effectiveness analysis. *British Medical Journal,* **312**, 1274–8.

12

....

Evaluating the dissemination of health promotion research

Gillian Lewando-Hundt and Salah Al Zaroo

The dissemination of health promotion research to policy-makers, practitioners, and users is essential if the gaps between research policy and practice are to be bridged. The findings of research are not the property of research scientists, the funders, or the respondents in the research. Rather, they are part of a shared body of knowledge which cumulatively leads to a better understanding of health promotion.

Despite its importance, research dissemination is often poorly resourced and not evaluated. There are papers arguing for dissemination and even arguing the importance of evaluating it (Green and Johnson 1996; Potvin 1996), but there are few published examples of evaluations. Without evidence of whether dissemination strategies of research are effective, it is likely that ineffective strategies will be pursued or effective strategies will be overlooked.

This chapter will begin by examining definitions of dissemination and will then look at how research is disseminated into policy, practice, and to users. The focus then moves on to an exploration of the barriers to dissemination and identifies ways of overcoming them, before finally discussing ways of evaluating dissemination.

Definitions of dissemination

Sometimes a differentiation is made between the processes of diffusion and dissemination, with diffusion defined as the spread of new knowledge to a defined population, via channels, over time, and dissemination defined as deliberate efforts to spread an innovation. Rogers (1983) however, views diffusion and dissemination as interchangeable terms. In this chapter we will define dissemination as follows:

'dissemination is about the communication of innovation, this being either a planned and systematic process or a passive and unplanned diffusion process'. (Crosswaite and Curtice 1991, p. 3)

Communication of knowledge through the dissemination of research findings is a key mechanism for the growth and development of a discipline. Health promotion is no exception to this. If anything the process of dissemination is more crucial to health promotion than other disciplines because of the guiding principles of participation, empowerment, and equity which underpin it.

Five types of transactions occur when disseminating research and information in relation to health promotion programmes (King *et al.* 1998). Such disseminating encourages:
1. information sharing about a new programme or finding;
2. support for the relevance of a new programme or policy;
3. decision making to adopt a new idea;
4. changing practices to implement a new idea or programme;
5. maintenance of a new practice or policy.

In evaluating dissemination we can distinguish between process evaluation, whereby the process of how and why these transactions occur, or do not occur, is traced, and outcome evaluation, which measures to what extent these changes are achieved. A further delineation can be made in terms of which arena the dissemination is being aimed at—policy, practice, or users.

Disseminating research into policy

There are four models which are generally referred to when discussing the dissemination of research to policymakers: the rational model; the limestone model; the gadfly model, and the insider model (Crosswaite and Curtice 1994). The **rational model** assumes that it is enough to make information available for it to be incorporated into policy making. This rarely, if ever happens. It is argued by others (Richardson *et al.* 1990) that research informs policy making indirectly and the **limestone model** is more often cited. This model postulates that research findings trickle down into policy making rather as water trickles down through porous limestone, circuitously and slowly. The **gadfly model** places as much emphasis on the dissemination of results as on the research itself, so there are meetings to feedback results to an advisory group, to the media, and to funders, and findings are published in a variety of reports and publications which address a range of audiences. Finally, the **insider model** operates when the researchers have links with those inside government or international and national agencies and are therefore able to adapt the presentation of research findings to address policy concerns.

Disseminating research into practice

The everyday practice of health professionals needs to be informed by research and yet effective ways of disseminating research to practitioners are not universally adopted. Continuing medical education has been examined in at least 50 randomized control trials, and there is evidence that it can improve physician performance (Davis *et al.* 1992). Continuing education to health professionals can take the form of:
- *Face to face interventions*: these include seminars, workshops, one to one supervisions.
- *Guidelines*: clinical guidelines are defined as systematically developed statements which assist in decisions on appropriate health care for specific conditions. There is evidence

that explicit guidelines improve clinical practice in almost all cases (Grimshaw and Russell 1993).

- *Newsletters*: these can be on tape, disc, or paper. For example The Safe Motherhood newsletter, funded by the World Health Organization, is distributed free in a variety of languages to practitioners in maternal health internationally.
- *The Internet*: evaluation of the use of the Internet for health promotion dissemination is in its infancy, but this will undoubtedly become an increasingly important source of information for professionals and practitioners.

Dissemination of research to subjects or service users

Users of services and community members have a right to be informed about research findings, particularly when they may have provided information for the research studies. This is a neglected area. Funding may be given for research but rarely for disseminating it to research subjects or service users. Also, career promotion is based on academic publications, not on the production and distribution of user friendly booklets and videotapes, or for speaking at public meetings.

The informed user can be a constructive influence on policy and practice. Today, research proposals to research councils in the UK or to the EC have to set out their strategies for dissemination and user engagement. This is a new and welcome development which should improve current practice. A recent study of how consumer organizations use health research information reported that, although they felt research was useful, they rarely read academic papers or reports but relied heavily on personal briefings by physicians or researchers (Glenton and Oxman 1998).

One mechanism to ensure some dissemination of research to users is the establishment of a consultative group for the coordination of the dissemination of findings. Consultation takes many forms and can be open and public, for example, in community meetings, or can be through nominated or elected committees. Dissemination to existing NGOs or community

---

Box 12.1 Participatory research in water and sanitation improvement: the development of the hygiene evaluation procedures (HEP) handbook

The HEP handbook was developed in response to practitioners' demand for guidelines on how to incorporate social and cultural considerations in the design of improved water supply, sanitation, and health promotion interventions. The handbook tackles the issue of participation of the researched by outlining three basic types of participation. Extractive participation (where researchers merely extract information and disappear) is discouraged in favour of consultative and interactive participation. Moreover, the methods/tools described in the handbook require the investigator to double-check and cross-check data by presenting it back to the study population for verification. In this way, their feedback on findings becomes part of the investigation process. This is a basic feedback mechanism to put in place if the final results are to be used by those concerned most, that is, the study population, whose practices health workers and others are trying to influence and change for the better.

The draft HEP handbook was field tested in different sites through consultative participation of intended users. Once in print, the dissemination process of the handbook and the approach it propagates have continued with seminars, talks, and training workshops for training of trainers. There is an evaluation sheet at the end of the book for users of the book to fill in. (Almedom *et al.* 1997)

---

groups is also a way of reaching a wider lay audience. This is time consuming, and sometimes delicate, but is worthwhile if research findings are to affect peoples' lives. The preparation of written information in local languages is often done. If such booklets are accompanied by meetings with community groups to discuss the material, then the dissemination will be more effective and the recommendations can be discussed and action plans formulated.

If a participative research approach is developed, with input from users at different stages of the research process, there is more likely to be an ownership of the research recommendations and results. The example in Box 12.1 illustrates this.

All too often outside researchers collect information from indigenous experts, publish academic papers which benefit their career, and fail to disseminate and share findings with the community that created these findings through their participation. This is an issue of research ethics concerning indigenous and users' rights to the knowledge and benefits of research which should be considered in all settings and regions.

Collaboration between researchers and subjects: action research

One strategy which takes cognizance of the important role of professional knowledge is practitioner-based research or action research with professionals and research scientists. Action research is problem-centred research bridging the gap between theory and practice. Unlike academic research, action research builds utilization strategies into overall research design. Involving professionals in practitioner-based action research also is an effective mechanism for ensuring the dissemination and acceptance of research findings. Others have called action research with professionals 'practitioner-based research'. There have been a number of studies undertaken by practitioners to establish the needs of users of their services and Box 12.2 gives two examples.

There are many further examples of action research which involve the active participation of practitioners (Hart and Bond 1995) and this model has much to offer. In addition, participatory action research with community members promotes a dialogue and interchange of knowledge between lay and professional bodies and can alter the basis of user involvement. Instead of users answering questions or being consulted about recommendations, the users involved in action research can frame the questions and the recommendations. This alters the power relations between researchers, professionals, and users and involves the dissemination of health promotion research findings within neighbourhoods and community groups. Community groups involved in action research are

---

> ## Box 12.2   Practitioner based action research in the field of learning difficulties
>
> A study in Coventry, England on the needs of people with learning difficulties involved a team of practitioners including a community psychiatric nurse, two social workers, two nursery nurses, and one translator of Asian languages. The professionals learnt how to carry out research and then presented their findings to management, to the families involved in the research, and to their colleagues. The project resulted in the establishment of a self help group for families and in some changes in policy and practice, such as regular benefit checks for families with children with learning difficulties.
>
> A similar study of the family needs of children with learning difficulties, with the team of a child development centre in southern Israel, resulted in the team advocating changes to the service they offered. They recommended, and partially implemented, integrated appointments, benefit checks, more focus on parental concerns, and more provision being given by Arabic speaking staff. (Lewando-Hundt *et al.* 1995)

often facilitated or aided by academics or health professionals and may be self-help groups or advocacy groups who have obtained funding for a specific project. A recent example is peer research conducted by Save the Children Fund with adolescent users of mental health services (Laws *et al.* 1999).

Barriers to dissemination

There are many barriers to timely dissemination and effective communication between researchers and users. These include:

- *Career structures*: academics may only get rewarded for publishing in peer reviewed journals; professionals may get no time for research or in-service training.
- *Institutional barriers*: funding may not resource dissemination and it may be difficult for academics, professionals, policymakers, and users to meet on neutral ground.

- *Ownership issues:* the funder may assert ownership of the results, or there may be copyright issues, so that the researcher may write the report but be unable to disseminate it to professionals or the community.
- *Delay of publishing in academic journals*: the process of submission, peer review, and re-submission can take up to eighteen months. This is often the period during which it would be appropriate to disseminate and yet the results are unpublished.
- *Technical barriers*: the language of research is technical and opaque. Dissemination requires clarity and simplicity of presentation both visually and verbally. Researchers are not trained in this (Crosswaite and Curtice 1994).

Overcoming barriers to dissemination

It is mistaken to view dissemination as a one-way traffic system of knowledge moving from researchers to implementers. It should be seen as a two-way process between researchers and implementers and the focus should be on mechanisms and linkages between the two groups (King *et al.* 1998). New knowledge belongs not to the scientists who develop it, but to everyone. Green (1987) argues for more efficient and systematic approaches to research dissemination aimed at the public. Knowledge is often the outcome of problem-solving activities by professionals; this knowledge is then reported by academics, and a closer relationship is needed to 'assume joint responsibility for knowledge creation, development and dissemination' (Eraut 1994, p. 57).

Ament (1994) proposed six strategies to overcome barriers to dissemination:

1. publishing in a variety of academic journals and publications that are read by policymakers;
2. presenting research papers at conferences attended by the policymakers and consumers;
3. presenting research findings to the groups who took part in studies;

4. using the mass media to publicize study findings; for example newspapers, radio, TV;
5. providing appropriate information to interest groups and lobbyists;
6. using personal contacts, formal, and informal networks for face-to-face meetings.

There have been several initiatives during the last ten years to narrow this gap, and the effective dissemination of research findings has become more of a priority both nationally and internationally. The recent trend to appoint more research liaison officers within universities and voluntary organizations is one strategy to strengthen linkages. Research liaison officers make links with funders, give advice on proposals, summarize studies, and network for the researchers or voluntary organization. These skills are not part of academic training. There is at least one international donor agency which uses a professional writer to train staff on how to present to politicians and prepare briefings (Dr M. Koblinsky, Mothercare International 1997, personal communication).

In addition to producing clear briefings on research findings to a variety of audiences using all types of media, it is often apposite to have advisory or steering groups whose membership reflects the constituencies the researchers wish to influence. Funders have recently placed more emphasis on dissemination, and many funding bodies request that researchers set out their dissemination strategies as part of their funding proposals. There is an increased willingness to fund these activities as part of the research. There is a recognition that dissemination is an integral part of all health promotion research activity and should be built into every programme, from initial stages through to completion. It is not an add-on activity.

Evaluating dissemination

Despite the considerable literature emphasizing the importance of dissemination and bemoaning the gap between research and practice, there has been little evaluation of the dissemination of health promotion programmes and what there has been does not have high visibility in the research field (King *et al.* 1998). Nevertheless there are some general issues and examples of good practice. Most of these involve developing linkages to bridge the gap between research and practice, and an evaluation of process as well as outcome.

A case study evaluating the dissemination of an information resource pack on key research findings and practice implications of a project on women's smoking in the UK (Blackburn *et al.* 1997) showed that, two years after the pack was distributed through professional and organizational networks, it was felt to have been useful to those that had requested it. This evaluation emphasized the importance of the user friendly approach in the form of cards, and the importance of using networks for distribution. It showed that if research based findings are presented appropriately for the target audience (in this case professionals) they are likely to use them.

The importance of linkage mechanisms and of attention to process is underlined by the failure of the Put Prevention into Practice (PHIP) programme which was developed to address barriers to prevention in family practice. After promoting the kit for two years through the Academy of Family Physicians in the US, only 27% of the members had heard about the programme. The availability of a kit was inadequate on its own and the researchers found a need for linkage mechanisms such as training, continuing medical education, and consultation services (Medder *et al.* 1997).

An example of successful dissemination of a health promotion programme through using linkages is the Canadian Heart Health Initiative which started as a programme in 1986 with the development of a policy framework and heart health surveys in ten provinces. Since 1989, all provinces have become involved in heart health demonstration programmes developed through setting up provincial heart health coalitions with between 15 and 40 community organizations. There were over 40 community interventions ongoing in 1996. Process evaluations of these interventions map 'the extent of community mobilization, leadership development,

coalition building, program acceptability and quality' (Stachenko 1996, p. S58). The outcome evaluation of these interventions looks at the impact of the programmes. The
dissemination phase will track the factors which influence
the wider transferability of these model interventions at a
local and regional level.

There is a need for more process evaluations of dissemination. Potvin (1996) advocates a pluralist approach to process
evaluation. This should include all stakeholders (professionals,
users, practitioners, policymakers, researchers) throughout
the evaluation process, so that multiple perspectives are included, strengthening the validity and reliability of the evaluation. Another means to ensure process evaluation which is
pluralistic and ongoing throughout a study is to set up advisory groups including all stakeholders (see Chapter 10).

Process and outcome evaluation of dissemination is a neglected area which must be developed so that effective dissemination can achieve the importance and visibility it
deserves. This type of evaluation is difficult to fund but recent
developments in health promotion research policy, emphasizing the need to develop evidence-based practice, may mean
more resources and the evaluation of dissemination strategies.
Dissemination is fundamental to the ethics and practice of
applied research in health promotion.

Key points

Effective dissemination can be encouraged by

- enhancing dialogue between researchers and users;
- developing practitioner-based or participatory action research;
- developing dissemination strategies from the beginning of the
  study.

Evaluation of dissemination requires

- a monitoring of both the process and outcomes using a range
  of methodologies;
- sufficient resourcing from the initial stages of the project.

Acknowledgements

We would like to thank Dr Astier Almedom for her contribution of the case study on the development of the Hygiene Evaluation Handbook and Dr Kathy Kahn for her comments on an earlier version of this chapter.

References

Almedom, A. M., Blumenthal, U., and Manderson, L. (1997). *Hygiene evaluation procedures: approaches and methods for assessing water and sanitation-related hygiene practices*. International Nutrition Foundation for Developing Countries (INFDC).

Ament, L. A. (1994). Strategies for dissemination of policy research. *Journal of Nurse-Midwifery*, **39**(5), 329–31.

Blackburn, C., Graham, H., and Scullion, P. (1997). Disseminating research finding on women's smoking to health practitioners: findings from an evaluation study. *Health Education Journal*, **56**, 113–24.

Crosswaite, C. and Curtice, L. (1991). *Dissemination of research for health promotion, a literature review*. Research Unit in Health and Behavioural Change, University of Edinburgh.

Crosswaite, C. and Curtice, L. (1994). Disseminating research results—the challenge of bridging the gap between health research and health action. *Health Promotion International*, **9**(4), 289–96.

Davis, D. A., Thompson, M. A., Oxman, A. D., and Haynes, B. (1992). Evidence of the effectiveness of the CME: a review of 50 randomized controlled trials. *Journal of the American Medical Association*, **268**, 1111–17.

Eraut, M. (1994). *Developing professional knowledge and competence*. Falmer Press, London and Washington.

Glenton, C. and Oxman, A. (1998). The use of evidence by health care user organizations. *Health Expectations*, **1**(1), 14–22.

Green, L. (1987). Three ways research influences policy and practice: the public's right to know and the scientist's responsibility to educate. *Health Education*, **18**, 44–9.

Green, L. W. and Johnson, J. L. (1996). Dissemination and utilization of health promotion and disease prevention knowledge: theory, research and experience. *Canadian Journal of Public Health*, **87**, Supplement 2, S11–17.

Grimshaw, J. M. and Russell, I. T. (1993). Effect of clinical guidelines on medical practice: a systematic review of rigorous evaluations. *Lancet*, **342**, 1317–22.

Hart, E. and Bond, M. (1995). *Action research for health and social care.* Open University Press, Buckingham.

King, L., Hawe, P., and Wise, M. (1998). Making dissemination a two-way process. *Health Promotion International*, **13**(3), 237–44.

Laws, S., Armitt, D., Metzendorf, W., Percival, P., and Reisel, J. (1999). *Time to listen: young people's experiences of mental health services.* Save the Children, London.

Lewando-Hundt, G., Porter, B., Faerman, M., Lubtzky, H., Goldshtein, E., Waternberg, M., *et al.* (1995). Moving towards a family oriented ethnic sensitive child development service. *Social Sciences in Health*, **1**(1), 45–59.

Medder, J., Sussman, J. L., Gilbert, C., Crabtree, B. F., McIlvain, H. E., McVea., K., *et al.* (1997). Dissemination and implementation of Put Prevention Into Family Practice. *American Journal of Preventive Medicine*, **13**(5), 345–51.

Potvin, L. (1996). Methodological challenges in evaluation of dissemination programs. *Canadian Journal of Public Health*, **87**, Supplement 2, S279–83.

Richardson, A., Jackson, C., and Sykes, W. (1990). Taking research seriously: means of improving and assessing the use and dissemination of research, HMSO, London.

Rogers, E. M. (1983). *Diffusion of innovations.* The Free Press, New York.

Stachenko, S. (1996). The Canadian health initiative: dissemination perspectives. *Canadian Journal of Public Health*, **87**, Supplement 2, S57–9.

13

Conclusions—integrating
methods for practice

Margaret Thorogood and Yolande Coombes

Health promotion has grown out of the mutual interest of
people from many disciplines in developing a new way of
thinking about health and ill-health. Ill-health is seen, not
merely as a collection of diseases for which biomedicine
should seek to find cures, but as a limitation to taking control
of one's life—which is why health promoters refer to 'health as
a resource for living' (see Chapter 1). In health promotion, the
biomedical and quantitative disciplines, using mechanistic
models of health, have met with the qualitative social
sciences, where health is viewed holistically, as an expression
of the relationship between an individual and the society in
which he or she lives. It is small wonder that health promotion
has been described as a 'Multi-disciplinary Tower of Babel'
(Kelleher 1999).

As the evaluation of health promotion comes of age, researchers from the different disciplines are coming to realize
that they are mutually interdependent. No method is better
than another: different methods address different dimensions
of what is meant by health. In this book we have attempted to

describe many of the wide range of methods which can be used in the evaluation of health promotion, as well as some of the problems which can arise. We did not intend that this book would comprise a complete enumeration of all the available methods, and, indeed, we doubt that any definitive list of such methods could be drawn up since new approaches are constantly being developed. However, we have aimed to discuss the most topical and important issues, which have bearing on the development and refinement of health promotion research and practice.

Discussions about the appropriate means to evaluate health promotion have a tendency to degenerate into heated but unproductive arguments, which have been well described by Ann Oakley (1998, p. 74):

'On the one side the social scientists align themselves with 'democratic' values and respect for the autonomy and subjectivity of lay people . . . castigating 'triallists' for their authoritarianism and denial of peoples liberty to choose . . . On the other side of the battle line, medical researchers may profess an inability to understand why qualitative research is relevant at all. . . . they are liable to complain that too much has been taken on trust, given the use of selective samples and the overriding importance of researchers interpretations.'

These battle lines are entirely negative in their effect, encouraging all those involved to strengthen and defend their position rather than to climb over the disciplinary walls and move toward new understandings. As Coombes argued in Chapter 3, health and health promotion are multi-faceted constructs, they need multi-disciplinary perspectives and methods to be understood. It is important that these approaches join forces to get closer to the 'truth' rather than continue to work in isolation.

Berridge's historical perspective provides an important reminder that new concepts of health promotion and of evidence-based practice are culturally defined, and sit within a historic tradition which can be traced back to the activities of Edwin Chadwick, who sought to reduce the burden of poverty by improving the health of the poor. Some of the most recent writers on health promotion have turned Chadwick's reasoning on its head, arguing that a reduction in the burden of ill-health can only be achieved by improving the economic conditions of the poorest people in society. Berridge also reminds us that the concept of evaluation itself is historically contingent on social processes.

The process of evaluation is contributing to the professionalization of health promotion and this, in itself, is a consequence of the emergence of evaluation as an acknowledged way of validating knowledge. Some disciplines, such as physics, have clear laws based on scientific experiment; other disciplines, such as anthropology, involve the validation of knowledge through discussion and debate from opposing epistemologies. Rigorous evaluation is crucial for health promotion to establish its disciplinary status, and a number of different methods will have to be used in this process.

The objectives of an intervention are the key criteria against which any evaluation must measure the outcome. Unfortunately, such criteria are not always used, either because the evaluation has not taken cognizance of the original objectives or because those objectives were not realistic or clearly defined at the outset. When an intervention is first being designed, the objectives should be stated and the evaluation methodology should be established. Part of the problem with evaluating health promotion is the need to evaluate the processes take place during an intervention. As Stewart points out, objectives often shift through the lifetime of a project or intervention. If adequate process evaluation is carried out, this need not be a problem and evaluation can then be tailored to the changing objectives. Evaluation must consider the formative and process stages of an intervention, and not just the outcome.

Florin and Basham describe the frustration of being unable to 'open the black box' and understand what actually goes on in the interaction between two people which forms the core of many health promotion interventions in clinical settings. Some of the severest critics of systematic reviews of health promotion have pointed out that insufficient attention has been paid to the nature of the interventions which are being reviewed (Speller *et al.* 1997). More work is urgently needed to develop agreed criteria to describe the content and theoretical basis of the interaction, in such a way that the intervention could be further tested by other researchers, or could be put into more general use. A greater attention to quality control is also needed. In many of the randomized controlled trials reported of health promotion in a clinical setting, not only has the description of the interaction been missing, but there is no attempt to monitor what actually did happen, as compared with what was intended to happen (See Chapter 4).

Other problems that arise with evaluation of health promotion interventions stem from uncertainty as to who we should consider as the recipients of the intervention we are evaluating. For example, as Jewkes points out, most of our interventions are aimed at the community, but do we really know who belongs to the community, and is it possible for us to define the community? Branigan and Mitchell remind us to be careful in selecting our research participants for qualitative research as the selection process can have a great impact on the results, and similarly Thorogood and Briton caution us that even randomized controlled trials may have more selection bias than is initially apparent. It is often important to separate the evaluator from the evaluated; often those that are carrying out an intervention also carry out the evaluation, but as Wellings and Macdowall suggest, this can mean that the evaluation lacks objectivity. Lewando-Hundt and Al-Zaroo remind us that the people we research or intervene with are joint owners of the results or new knowledge, and that dissemination is therefore an ethical obligation. If health promotion is to grow as a discipline the importance of dissemination can not be underestimated.

We have highlighted some of the problems associated with defining the content of interventions, but problems also arise from being unable to predict what may happen in the more distant future. As Naidoo shows, simulation models can offer a way forward, while Wonderling and Karnon show how economic evaluation can allow us to compare several potential interventions. The results of process evaluations or the evaluation of proximal outcomes can often be as informative as a formal evaluation of more distal outcomes. However, health promotion interventions will have to find new and creative ways of bridging the time gap between the intervention and the outcome (where the outcome is measurable).

It is apparent from this book that, as health promotion develops into a mature discipline, it will need a combination of approaches to evaluation using a variety of methods. Neither qualitative or quantitative approaches should be considered easier nor, conversely, more rigorous than the other. Nor should one approach be considered the exclusive domain of one group of researchers. Social scientists are capable of learning how to carry out epidemiological investigations and biomedical researchers can learn how to carry out a qualitative interview. What is essential is that methods are used appropriately for the job in hand and are used to evaluate those areas of health promotion activity where they are most able to increase our knowledge and evidence base. Each evaluation and health promotion intervention must be assessed on its own merits. It is not possible to compare within a universal framework evaluations which use different methodologies. Multi-disciplinary or combined interventions that are being developed should be further enhanced, as there is no single theory or methodological approach for the evaluation of health promotion.

Key points

- High quality evaluation of health promotion is essential. Evaluation should be designed at the same time that the intervention is planned, and adequate resources should be allocated.

- Effective evaluation of health promotion interventions and programmes requires a multi-method approach. No one method or theory is adequate.

- As a new and expanding discipline, health promotion needs to establish a strong evidence base, which can only be done through accurate, reliable, and valid methods of evaluation.

References

Kelleher, C. (1999). Evaluating health promotion in four key settings. In *Health promotion striving for certainties* (ed. J. K. Davies and G. MacDonald), pp. 47–67. Routledge, London.

Oakley, A. (1998). Experimentation in social science: the case of health promotion. *Social Sciences in Health*, **4**(2) , 73–89.

Speller, V., Learmonth, A., and Harrison, D. (1997). The search for evidence of effective health promotion. *British Medical Journal*, **315**, 361–2.

Index

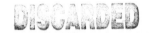